C0-BQB-591

THE HEART MACHINE

By the same author

MARGARET

DOROTHY: A portrait

THE RACE BEFORE US

CLARE

The Heart Machine

A Personal Account of Open-Heart Surgery

JAMES DAVIDSON ROSS

TAPLINGER PUBLISHING CO., INC.
New York

First published in the United States in 1973 by
TAPLINGER PUBLISHING CO., INC.
New York, New York

Printed in Great Britain

Library of Congress Catalog Card Number: 73-6183

ISBN 0-8008-3821-1

CONTENTS

FOREWORD BY E. W. B. CARDIFF, Director General of the British Heart Foundation Appeal *page* vii

1 Introducing a heart 1

2 The woman in the case 9

3 Rumblings 25

4 Hobson's Choice 41

5 Decisions 58

6 Countdown 72

7 Razor's edge 92

8 Out of the valley 102

9 The X-factor 116

10 Hearts are trumps 128

Post (Op) Script 141

FOREWORD

TWELVE years ago all Mr Ross's courage, stamina and faith could not have kept him alive.

Today, the skill of the cardiac team, the surgeons, the nurses, the technicians and the advances of cardiac operative techniques have made open heart surgery in this country a successful routine operation, especially when there are not the added disabilities from which Mr Ross suffered.

It must be a great comfort to heart sufferers to know that this operation and other treatment made possible by the increase in both knowledge and skill are now available in many Cardiac Centres throughout the British Isles where progress has more than kept pace with the rest of the world.

E. B. W. CARDIFF

AUTHOR'S NOTE

In the following pages I have suppressed or altered the real names of all surgeons, doctors, nurses or technical staff of any of the hospitals which had to put up with me as one of their patients during 1971. I have done this in deference to the etiquette of our medical services which demands anonymity for its members. If, however, any of those over-worked, under-paid heroes recognises him or herself in this narrative, then I make no apology.

Dedications of books are sometimes strictly formal.
This one is not.
I give it, from the depths of a mended heart, to
Johanna, my wife,
Pat and Christopher, our strength,
the medical, nursing and technical staff of the
Walsgrave Hospital,
and a cardiac surgeon who must remain anonymous,
but without whom this book would never have been
written.

The wind was against them now, and Piglet's ears streamed behind him like banners as he fought his way along, and it seemed hours before he got them into the shelter of the Hundred Acre Wood and they stood up straight again, to listen, a little nervously, to the roaring of the gale among the treetops.

'Supposing a tree fell down, Pooh, when we were underneath it?'

'Supposing it didn't', said Pooh after careful thought.

From *The House at Pooh Corner* by A. A. Milne; quoted by kind permission of C. R. Milne and Methuen & Co. Ltd.

I

INTRODUCING A HEART

The overhead spotlight died, and the grey face of the monitoring screen glowed, broke up, then steadied. The sharply etched casing of a man's ribs showed up in the dim theatre; behind them the vague lump of a beating human heart. And then, snaking up from the left-hand corner of the picture, appeared a tube, a dark filament of shadow—feeling, probing, crawling across the interior of the chest. To hover over the top of the heart; to pause; to plunge down gingerly into the blob of the living muscle.

With an effort I pulled my hypnotised gaze away from the screen, avoided the wildly swinging blip on the oscilloscope—I didn't need to see that to know my heart was objecting—and cocked an eye at the nurse standing by my head.

'Science fiction!' I stated firmly.

'No—just science. Is it hurting you?'

Well, was it? I glanced down my prone body; at the X-ray camera squatting over my chest, at my outstretched right arm—bloody, tube-infested, and presided over by two green-gowned doctors who muttered gibberish while poking and pulling at the open incisions—only one glance at that, then a hasty shift to the silent, masked and gowned figures standing round the small theatre; at the mass of X-ray equipment, electronic equipment, surgical equipment; at that paralysing monitor, at the senior radiological sister standing at my feet watching me all the time with steady, all-seeing eyes. Was it hurting?

'No. Just—peculiar. I'd rather it was you here than me.'

She laughed. 'Snap! I don't want it. Are you comfortable?'

'No. Darned uncomfortable. How far have we got? Isn't it about time you threw me out?'

She eased my head on the table, her hand supporting my aching neck. 'We're about half-way there. Just hang on, we'll be as quick as we can.'

Half-way there: for the love of mike! The clock high up on the wall of the theatre told me I had already been more than an hour on that unmentionable table: another hour of—this. I looked into the impassive face of the X-ray tube and tried to think myself elsewhere. Tried not to watch the catheter wriggling around inside my heart. Tried to pray, then decided to leave that one to others less immediately involved. Tried to picture where all this was leading to. And found myself back at the monitoring screen, watching the probes, feeling, being. Another hour: good grief!

They had told me precisely what was to happen, and I hadn't liked the sound of it. But it was necessary. Too right it was! There is a limit to how long the human heart can go on operating with two of its valves almost completely out of action. And I knew I had nearly reached that limit—after all, they had kept going for thirty years, which was precisely thirty years longer than anyone had expected them to. But now the crunch had come: either those incompetent, calcified, leaking bits of muscle in my heart must be replaced, or I might as well start composing my swan-song.

'Yes, some tests', the cardiologist had said a few weeks before. 'Absolutely necessary before we can even begin to talk about operating. I want to have you in hospital for a while, and carry out what we call a cardiac catheterisation. Heard of it?'

'No, but I know what catheters are.' And disliked what I knew. Thirty years previously during a mammoth stay in hospital, after I had collapsed with a king-sized attack of bacterial endocarditis, I had known many of my fellow patients submit to catheters—and always in the same area, it seemed. Catheters had meant tubes being shoved into intensely personal parts of one's body, and I had always been thankful that I was the possessor of a cock-eyed heart, not a kidney or bladder on the blink. 'What do you mean—cardiac catheterisation?' I asked suspiciously, 'You can't poke catheters into a heart.'

The cardiologist had tapped my chest thoughtfully. 'That is precisely what we can do. We make an incision over a certain artery and vein in your arm, and pass a tube—a catheter—up into your chest and so into every chamber of your heart. By that means we are able to measure valve leakage, oxygen saturation, and so on. And obtain the sort of X-rays we couldn't otherwise get.'

'How?' Still suspiciously.

He had grinned amicably at me. 'At a certain point in the proceedings we—ah, squirt a type of iodine directly into your heart and take a series of X-rays. We finish up with a very good working blue-print of your heart', he had finished blandly.

'Charming! It doesn't sound my idea of a pleasant indoor game. Is it absolutely necessary?'

'Absolutely.' The devil of it was that I knew he was right. Thirty-one years ago, a young and very fit member of the RAF, I had developed rheumatic fever, endocarditis, valvular disease of the heart and God-knows what-all complications which had kept me on my back in hospital for two and a half years. No one had expected me to survive—there were none of the modern antibiotics or drugs to cope with that sort of devastation in 1940—but survive I had, due partly to the constitution of an elephant, partly to first-class nursing, and generally to a certain bloody-mindedness which has usually stood me in good stead.[1]

[1] See *The Race Before Us* by James D. Ross (Hodder & Stoughton).

Not only survived but gone on to live the next thirty years fully and vigorously. Down those years various doctors had removed their stethoscopes from shocked ears and warned me that unless I slowed right down—indeed, led the life of a complete invalid—I was bound to die fairly immediately from acute heart failure.

I had ignored the lot of them. Worked hard, lived hard, and, during the first decade of that period, smoked and drank decidedly too hard. Always in the background, generally unobtrusive, sometimes clamouring its protest, was my heart: the mitral valve, as I was repeatedly told, 'leaking like a sieve', the aortic incompetent, sloshing blood everywhere but in the right direction, and gradually calcifying into uselessness. Twice during those thirty years it took outraged strike action. The first time in 1959 when a full-blown failure laid me on my back for a month; the second in 1964 when I developed pneumonia following a brisk attack of flu, and my heart decided it didn't like it.

But apart from that it had kept going. A nuisance, tiresomely restrictive at times, always with that fluctuating niggle of pain in the left breast—but working.

I had married in 1946 (amid the grave doubts of the doctors), and lived seventeen tremendous years with a woman in a million until, with appalling suddenness, she fell down and died from one massive attack of coronary thrombosis at the age of thirty-eight.[1] And still my own battered heart went on working.

For a dreary, grey period I led the life of a widower, then to my great surprise met a second woman in a million and married again. At the ripe age of forty, with a thoroughly unserviceable heart, and by now becoming badly crippled with spondylitis and osteoarthritis (the old, old legacy from rheumatic fever), I found myself married to a girl sixteen

[1] See *Clare* by James D. Ross (Hodder & Stoughton).

years my junior, and, there being nothing wrong with my hormones, in due time the immensely proud and besotted father of two children.

And still that tough bit of muscle I call a heart kept going.

It kept going through five years in which I edited a small newspaper, working every hour the good God had given me, plus a few more it sometimes seemed, until the paper folded under the economic pressures bearing down on most newspapers nowadays. It kept going through the hard slog of free-lance journalism, of climbing mountains in Wales with my small son; of living, working and playing to the maximum. By the beginning of 1971 I had achieved the free-lance writer's dream: several hard and fast contracts to bring in the bread and butter, with a growing number of the acceptances of the work which I wanted to do. I felt fit, alert and active; my days (and evenings) full of work, the future bright and promising. True, my arthritic hip had become such a nuisance that I had visited an orthopaedic surgeon and been offered a brand-new artificial hip—if a certain cardiologist agreed that my heart could stand the operation. So optimistic was I that I had no doubt that within a few months I would get that hip, and after years of walking like a lop-sided crab would be as sprightly as any father of a five-year-old son could wish to be.

Such was my state of mind and being in February 1971. I really should have known better. Thirty years is a long time for a ropey heart to keep going, even if it is given a modicum of consideration. And mine had merely been told to get on with its work. The hot-line between my worn-out valves and nemesis must have been sizzling.

The cardiologist who should have passed judgement on my hip, and hadn't, straightened up from my arm and smiled at me. 'All right?' he asked.

I tore my gaze away from the monitoring screen and slewed my head round to him. 'You're making a bloody mess of my arm—literally!' I said nastily.

'You'll be surprised how good we are at mopping up blood. Now look, we are going to take two series of twenty X-rays each, and while they are being shot we're going to put this iodine into you. You'll feel a sort of hot sensation spreading out from your chest very rapidly—bit unpleasant, I'm afraid, and it will probably leave you with a headache, but it doesn't take very long.'

'And be prepared for a lot of noise while the X-rays are being taken', said the nurse at my head. 'It goes off like a gun—bang, bang, bang—very rapidly. Twenty times, in fact. But it's quite quick.'

I watched while they hauled my unfeeling right arm above my head and swung a camera in towards the side of my chest. For goodness sake, how much longer would this go on? Nearly two hours now. Two hours of my arthritic bones seizing up on this wretched table; of blood and tubes and now high-grade ink being squirted into me; of unpleasant feelings and worse imaginings and, possibly worst of all, a growing exhaustion which was becoming increasingly difficult to combat. And I had an itch on my bottom I couldn't even scratch.

'O.K. Get on with it then', I muttered.

An incendiary bomb exploded inside me as the iodine flooded into my heart and the X-rays went off like a machine-gun. An extraordinary sensation of heat swept outwards through my entire body, flooding out to fingers, toes, even hair. A little man with a pneumatic drill started a sharp tattoo inside my skull, and a rash of sweat broke out all down my prostrate form.

'Good God, are you trying to induce the change of life?' I asked breathlessly—'Talk about hot flushes!'

'Once more and it's done.' A second camera came down onto my chest, a second dose of liquid dynamite shot through the tubes to my heart, and again the incendiary went off. I blinked, rolling my head to try and avoid the pneumatic drill.

'All finished,' announced the cardiologist, 'We'll sew you up, then back to your ward and you can rest.' He looked at me quizzically over my outstretched arm as his assistant wound in what seemed like several yards of bloodied tubing. 'Was it too unpleasant?'

'I could do with a beer', I countered.

'No beer today—have one tomorrow. No food until this evening and no hopping out of bed for twenty-four hours.'

The X-ray sister slid a pillow under my head as the assistant cardiologist ploughed in with needle and catgut. 'Where did you get that tan? she asked.

'Wales. I came straight back from holiday into hospital—I ask you!'

'But it's not stopped raining for a month.'

'We had sunshine continuously for eleven days,' I stated firmly, 'You know—it shines on the righteous.'

'And were you righteous?' asked the cardiologist. Was it a holiday, or did you climb Cader again?'

'Er—not Cader.'

'But you did some climbing?'

'A very modest pimple.' I watched the plaster being strapped round my arm and wondered what it would feel like when it returned to life. 'If you really want to know I went bathing every day.'

'You went in the sea?'

'Yes.'

'And may I ask what your valves thought about that little activity?' he enquired politely.

'They were all right. Anyway, they had to lump it.' I dropped the subject hastily. 'When will you know about the operation, Doctor. How long does it take to sort out this morning's effort?'

'Someone is going to be very busy this evening working out the most complicated mathematics, and I'll be able to let you know what we advise on Thursday.'

And it was Monday now. Three more days before I came to the moment of truth. Not that there were many doubts in my mind. If I had the operation there was at least a chance. Without it there was none.

2

THE WOMAN IN THE CASE

THE thirty years co-operation from my heart had ended abruptly one Sunday evening in February 1971.

I had had a good day. Church in the morning with my family (a discipline we not only subscribe to but enjoy); a couple of pints of best bitter at midday; a couple of hours sleep in the afternoon; two more hours entertaining the children followed by a sort-out at my desk for the next day's work; and later, following an early supper and bath, I wandered downstairs in pyjamas and dressing gown to watch the latest BBC production of one of our treasured classics. Lord knows which, the events of the next few hours wiped that from my mind most effectively.

And I felt fit! I had scarcely given my heart a thought in months. Why should I? It was bumping and banging along as usual, and if it seemed to be racing a lot then there was nothing surprising in that. For weeks the country had been gripped by a postal strike, and, added to my normal quota of work, I had been driving many hundreds of extra miles to deliver copy demanded on deadlines. I knew I had been overdoing it, but that was nothing new. Rather was it the norm.

Out of the blue, the room, the television set, my wife Johanna, the cat sprawled on my lap—all tilted and went dark. They reappeared out of a haze of dizziness, and for a long time I sat still, trying to work out what was happening. Waves of heat were flowing over me, and my heart had suddenly started beating a tattoo which would not have disgraced a pop drummer. At the slightest movement I felt I was falling backwards, the crazily tilting room offending my vision with its see-saw gyrations.

Then out of the confusion came an old, old feeling I had not known for several years: the consciousness and awareness of death stepping out of the wings. And waiting.

At last I managed to speak through the immense weariness which was falling on me, blotting out all other thoughts and emotions.

'Jo, I'm feeling odd.'

She was round in a flash. 'I thought you didn't like the play—Jim, what is it? Is it your heart?'

I nodded, almost beyond speech. The gallop under my ribs had stepped up a notch; it felt as though some wild crazed creature was trapped inside, struggling frantically to get loose. With every movement an impossible burden I managed to push myself to my feet, and somehow—God alone knows how—Johanna half pushed, half carried me to bed. And death, who had been my companion so often thirty years before, drifted into the bedroom after me. And waited.

Such a common crisis! Nowadays it hits scores of thousands of households in our country every year. And although for the person suffering the attack—coronary, paroxysm or what-have-you—the episode is unpleasant and can be fantastically painful, it is something which narrows horizons and leaves him or her with the solitary, and very basic problem of survival. It is far, far more traumatic, far greater an ordeal for the partner, husband or wife, who has to watch, and endure, and cope.

When Johanna married me in 1964 she knew I had a badly diseased heart. She knew I had had valvular disease for longer than she had lived, and with eyes wide open she had gone into a marriage which she realised could end abruptly at any time. Such is the way of many women. They are, on the whole, far greater realists than men, and reckon (rightly) that a year, or a month, even a day or an hour of happiness, more than compensates for the risk of future tragedy. Most women are much less obsessed with the future than men: they prefer to live and love and suffer, if need be, in the present, and their lives are the richer for their philosophy.

Nevertheless, it cannot be easy to take on someone in marriage for whom, according to all the medical rules, time has long since run out. And that is precisely what Johanna did. She married a widower sixteen years older than herself whom the experts said could not survive, and for nearly seven years she lived with the daily knowledge that this day—today—now—could be the finale to her happiness and security. Thus, although this book is to be about the miracle of how a cardiac surgeon chopped into my battered heart, and, against odds of more than fifty per cent likelihood of failure, gave me an incredible new lease of life (at least, I trust that will be the outcome: as I write I have not yet had the operation), despite that central drama this book must also be about a woman. And her ability and faith which enabled her to ride with confidence one hell of a year of crisis, anxiety and fear.

Despite her name Johanna is a Londoner. With decent heels she just about touches five feet; her hair has enough red in it to make one wary of pushing one's luck; and her figure (after having two babies) remains that of a ballet dancer—which she was, until circumstances and ill-health forced her to drop a budding career. She has the energy of a high-grade dynamo; an intelligence and independence which make the womens' lib movement look old hat—while surrendering not a milligramme of her femininity; and she can sink a pint of Double Diamond at a speed not to be despised by a thirsty docker.

I met her when she was twenty-four years old and working in a Bond Street store. But it was a long way from London's

West End that I first laid my jaded eyes on her. I say jaded deliberately, and it understates the case.

When my first wife, Clare, died, I was the Warden of the Coventry Diocesan Retreat and Conference House—which meant, in effect, that I was running a specialised small hotel with clerical and spiritual complications. And doing that kind of job with a chronic shortage of staff, twelve hours (at least) solid work each day, and a decidedly fifth-rate body, is no joke. For a year after Clare's death I buried myself in work, with all my hard-pressed systems at go, but by the summer of 1964 I knew I had to take a holiday or become a casualty myself.

After a year of widowerhood and work I had had it! I felt stifled, hemmed in, restricted, and I just had to get away from everything. But where to go? I was sick to death of people, but afraid of solitude: where to go and find company if I wanted it, but where I could also escape and be on my own if I wished? For weeks I dithered, and I am not a ditherer by nature. I loathe indecision. Finally I decided to go to Lee Abbey in Devonshire: I had been there half a dozen times in the past, knew and liked the place and people, loved the north Devon coast and countryside.

Lee Abbey is a Christian holiday centre run by a community of (mostly) young lay men and women. It is evangelistic in concept, liberal in practice, and over the past twenty years has been a haven for many thousands seeking help or peace or inspiration amid the storms of life. The house, taking well over a hundred guests, lies in its own widespread, and unspoilt grounds a couple of miles west of Lynton on the north Devon coast. Clare and I had first gone there in 1957, somewhat nervously, alarmed at the thought that we might be putting our heads into some sort of evangelistic noose. We could not have been more wrong. Evangelism, of course, was there. It could not be otherwise when the forty or fifty members of the community were doing their best to live, not just talk, but live, by the finest precepts which Christ ever propounded. But they rammed nothing down our wary throats, got at us over nothing, and we enjoyed one of the best holidays we had ever known. So we had gone back there, again and again. Now I booked to go once more, but not quite certain if I was being wise in doing so. I was putting myself into a position where I would have to mix with, and be civilised to a lot of people, and after the past year of flat-out work with hundreds of people I was too tired even to want to make the effort of just being with people. Yet, if I went away with friends I was being an appendage. If I went off to some solitary spot I would quite likely become downright morbid. After going round in circles for weeks I threw my cases in the boot of my car and set off for Devon. I found I was not the only person engaged in this pastime: I had forgotten it was a Saturday in mid-August, and the whole world and his wife, plus car and kids, was on the roads leading to the west of England.

Several hot, crawling, reeking hours later I dropped out of the monster charging down the road to Minehead and sought refuge, food and gin and tonic in a wayside pub. Sitting watching the endless traffic go by, the whole indecision of the last few months seemed to crowd into the moment: why in the name of wonder was I spending weary hours driving to a place to which I didn't really want to go, to become one of a hoard of people talking interminably about religion and churchy things of which, in any case, I was sick to death? Why not pull out of this stupid, sheeplike crowd of holiday-makers and go—Oh, damn it, anywhere! Fed up to the teeth with myself and the crowd around me I swallowed my gin, tramped back to the car, and got on the road to Devon again. To this day I don't know why: I did not want to go, and I have often wondered what would have happened if I had turned the car round and just run off into the blue—but I lacked the will to do anything which demanded initiative. I shoved my car back into the juggernaut, and headed towards Lynton.

For better or for worse, and just fourteen months after Clare's death, I arrived at Lee Abbey.

From my eyrie high on the cliffs I gazed out over the sunlit Bristol Channel and reviewed the past forty-eight hours. I came to the conclusion that I had not been exactly sociable. Lee Abbey had been as casually informal and welcoming as ever, but I had avoided close contact with my fellow-guests as much as possible, getting out to the wind-swept loneliness of Exmoor for most of the day and using the house as little more than a nightly lodging place. True, Lee Abbey was working its usual spell on me and I was already clambering out of the unfamiliar rut of introspection along which I had been wandering for too long. But people, parties, invitations, talks, all the complexity of activities which are so much a part of a Lee Abbey holiday, I was avoiding like the plague. Nevertheless, the peace of the house was filtering into me, and still carrying that peace I would drive off into the depths of the moors near Simonsbath, or turn down towards the Doone Valley and spend the day alone in a haze akin to pantheism. Now I had retired to a spot I had discovered some years earlier when I had been among a crowd of holiday-makers who had fought a severe cliff-fire endangering Lee Abbey. During that fire in 1959, when heath fires had devastated many thousands of acres in south and west England, the cliffs from Lee Bay eastwards into the Valley of the Rocks had been denuded of nearly all foliage. In the continuing dry weather, and hampered by an acute water shortage, the community of Lee Abbey had organised a continuous fire-watch around the cliffs, made up of community members and guests: the house had been threatened once and they did not want it to happen again. Clare and I had done our stint on the cliff top near the famed (and legendary) Jennifred's Leap, and, seeing smoke puff up from the scorched face of the cliff, had slithered down to investigate, at considerable risk to life and limb. The small smouldering area was dealt with easily, but hunting around for the best way back to the cliff top we found a blackened rocky track leading off beneath an overhang in the cliff. Crawling round it like flies on a wall we came out eventually on a small ledge which was completely concealed from above, with only sheer cliffs below and the Bristol Channel stretching out to the dim and distant shore-line of Wales. It was easy to see that, with the cliff covered in its usual heavy mantle of foliage, this eyrie had been quite invisible and probably unknown to the thousands of holiday-makers who roamed round these cliffs each summer. We made a mental note of the approaches to it, marking it down as a superb retreat from the maddening crowd on any future visits to this corner of Devon.

As events turned out Clare never again risked her neck on that crazy track, but I did. Armed with a couple of bottles of beer, sandwiches and chocolate, writing materials and a book, I left the house immediately after breakfast that day in 1964 and hot-footed it to the top of the cliffs. It took a good hour to find the spot on the edge over which Clare and I had descended to fight our small fire five years earlier—the fire seemed to have encouraged even more luxuriant growth, providing excellent camouflage for land-marks, and, in any case, my memory had grown vague. But find it I did, and for the whole of that day, suspended between cloudless sky and unrippled sea, I neither heard nor saw the faintest sign that any other human being inhabited this planet. It was a time outside time: a moment, though I did not realise it, between the old and the new. Without even being aware of it, I had crossed the lowlands. I was up in the hills again, only hours separating me from a new chapter of this odd business we call life.

I watched her hesitating by the door, obviously taken aback by the tumult which always filled the dining-room at meal times: she was a new guest, nervous, advancing with an effort into a sea of well over a hundred faces, none of which she knew, into a situation which was strange and daunting. She walked diffidently between the rowdy tables, searching for a vacant seat, and sank down hurriedly into the only one available—opposite me. I grinned at her sardonically.

'Serves you right for being three days late for the party.'

'I couldn't get away before. Is it always like this?'

'Always. Sometimes more so. You'll get used to it, and the grub's acceptable.'

'You've been here before?'

'I practically have shares in the place.'

'Do you like it? I mean, I've only heard . . . . '

'I know: evangelism and Are You Saved, brother—sister, rather. Don't take any notice, the place is all right. Nobody is going to get at you.'

Eyebrows raised under reddish-brown hair, and a very direct look shot across the table at me: 'Except you, perhaps?'

'What do you mean—except me?'

'Well, are you always so brusque?'

'Always. Why have you come here?'

'I've been ill and I wanted a holiday.'

'Well, you've put your foot in it properly! You'll be worked to death here and stay up half the night talking to a shower of Christians. You'll go back a wreck.'

'Thank you. I seem to have made a good start.'

That was the Tuesday. On Wednesday, dining-room and

redheads forgotten, I went over to Hunters Inn five miles down the coast for a drink and a spot of male companionship. The weather continued fine, the time slipped by, and I continued unwinding. Thursday evening saw me giving a talk to the guests in the lounge during the evening's Epilogue—one of the penalties (or privileges, I can never make up my mind which) of writing books which grip the public imagination. I spoke about the death from cancer of my young sister-in-law, Margaret, at the age of fifteen a few years previously, and how this unlikely event had turned me into a Christian. Afterwards, as I walked out of the lounge to get a cup of coffee, there came a rush of feet behind me, my arm was grasped, and I found myself looking into the flushed face of the late-arrival of Tuesday evening.

'You're Jim Ross. You wrote the book *Margaret*!' she burst out. 'I've heard people saying the author of *Margaret* was here, but I had no idea it was you!'

'Um—yes.'

'I'm so glad! You don't know how glad I am to meet you', she said simply.

'Um—yes', I repeated, and fled.

So Friday came, and I continued on my (by now mildly) anti-social course. But Lee Abbey was working its old familiar magic on me, and I did not escape to the moors directly I had eaten my breakfast. Instead I stayed close to the house, faintly aware that I was waiting for something to happen, but without any idea what it would be. Late afternoon found me sitting on the terrace overlooking the broad sweep of Lee Bay round to the promontory of Woody Bay; below on the beach tiny figures ran and lay and swam; behind me an agreeable sound of tea-cups served as a reminder that lunch was a long way in the past and supper several hours in the future. It was all very lazy, and the Retreat House seemed a million miles away.

A figure appeared on the cliff path down from Jennifred's Leap, and moved with swinging stride towards the terrace. As she drew level with me she hesitated fractionally, then with one swift, uncertain glance in my direction walked on past. I listened to her retreating footsteps, and for an eternal moment while the world paused, the sun-filled view was etched deep into my memory. I swung round in my seat.

'You look as though you've walked miles', I called out, 'And it's much too hot. I, on the other hand, have spent the afternoon contemplating . . . '

'Sleeping?'

'Contemplating the view! Let me get you some tea.'

She lay back in the chair beside me and accepted a cigarette. 'Thanks, I'd love some. Don't you think it's time you asked my name?'

'Yes. What is your name?'

'Johanna.'

'Well, Joanna . . . '

'Johanna! It's got an 'h' in it. It's German I think, although I'm a Londoner.'

'Then why the German name?'

'I haven't the faintest idea—but I do know I'm dying for that tea.'

Dodging back with a laden tea-tray to our seats on the terrace, I watched the small figure waiting for me. She gazed back with steady eyes as I spread the tea around us. 'You snubbed me the other night', she declared flatly.

'I'm not snubbing you now.' I glanced at her cautiously: 'What are you doing this evening?'

'Nothing.'

'Good—let's do it together.'

We spent the whole evening together, and that was the start of it. I did not sleep easily that night. Doubts, fears, panic almost, at the thought that I was getting far too friendly with a complete stranger, sixteen years my junior, jostled round my head. I told myself a hundred times that it was merely one of those casual holiday friendships which grow in a few hours, and die as quickly, but deep inside I didn't believe it. I had met many girls and women in the grey period since Clare died, and nothing but the most platonic thoughts had ever entered my mind. But now? A heart-shaped face, red-brown hair and a pair of hazel eyes filtered through my dreams when eventually I drifted off to sleep. Plato was dropping rapidly in the charts, Venus already heading for the top.

So began a period when I tried my damndest to run full tilt in two diametrically opposed directions. Johanna and I were attracted to each other powerfully from the word go—mentally, physically, spiritually. We shared much in common, as we found out in the dream-like days which followed. Our Christian faith, our critical views on the Church, our tastes in music, art, books, our sense of humour—all were common ground, and for myself, emerging from my self-imposed anti-social period, it was like coming upon an oasis in the middle of a particularly arid desert. We spent the rest of that holiday in one another's company, weaving a tapestry of companionship against those sunlit days which rapidly deepened into love —and keeping zip-fasteners tightly drawn across our lips against any such dangerous subject.

Because mentally I was running like a mad thing. My thoughts became a racing whirlpool as one part of me strove to move forward while the other part cried 'stay!' Stay where you are in the grey lowlands, where no decisions are needed, where no loyalties are called in question, where you will not have to be challenged by the realities of life and living. Oh, those loyalties, and how muddled one can get! How much those of us who are living cling to the dead, striving to impose on that which is now wholly spiritual that which is very human and material. How worried I was about what Clare would be thinking of me now! How agonized that she would consider I was betraying her, or her memory! How frantically I tried to recall the face of the dead Clare, and saw only the smiling face of the living Johanna.

What a state we do get ourselves into at times to be sure!

Deliberately I kept all conversation, all contact with Johanna on a light level, but equally deliberately I sought out her company for every possible minute of the day. And she did not run. The fact that I was forty years old to her twenty-four, a cripple—Oh yes, let me use a word I loathe—a cripple with a pretty ropey expectancy of life: none of it seemed to matter to her at all. Indeed, she did not even seem to notice these things. Day followed golden day and the thread between us tightened. I resolved it must come to a head before the holiday ended. Anything else was dishonest. I made a date to take her out on the moors on the Thursday afternoon before we were due to return to our respective homes. One way or another we had to have this thing out.

Driving through Malmsmead I ran the car off the road short of Oaresford and we lit cigarettes, gazing out over the long steep valley of Badgworthy Water. We were deep in Doone country, and ever since a child the fascination of this corner of England had gripped me: I must admit that I am a romantic, and the ghost of Jan Ridd must live in the heart of all who confess to romanticism. I had not chosen the setting deliberately, but it certainly fitted the mood.

'Johanna, you're going back to London tomorrow, and I'm leaving on Saturday; I think there are certain things that have got to be said.'

She nodded, silent, gazing out over the sun-drenched landscape. I ground out my cigarette and took a deep breath.

'Jo, I'm a widower, and I loved my wife very deeply. I'm

also forty, sixteen years older than you. I'm lame, I've got a lousy heart, and there's not a doctor in the world who would guarantee my future. I've got about tuppence-halfpenny to my name, and I'm seriously considering quitting my job.' Swinging round I clasped her arms and made her look at me: 'I'm also quite hopelessly in love with you and getting more so every day. What are we going to do about it?'

She did not answer in words, but that first kiss took both of us beyond the lowlands and into a new life which stood waiting only to be grasped.

In a dream we wandered over the moor, exploring hamlets and valleys with the delight of children who have discovered a new world. In a dream we returned at last to Lee Abbey and somehow got through an evening of people and events who only impinged vaguely on the periphery of our reality. And at length, in mutual silence and consent, we went upstairs to the chapel and became part of the stillness.

How long we stayed there I do not know, only that it was several hours. Each of us was facing the future—Johanna serenely, myself in a renewed agony of indecision. We knew we loved one another, but further than that—what? Marriage? The word had not even been mentioned: events were going too swiftly, time was rushing us along so fast that neither of us could yet have grasped the implications of this explosive relationship. At some point she left me in the dimness of the chapel: she had faced her future with what I was to discover was characteristic courage, and had accepted it. She knew I must do the same and decide my future one way or another, and she knew I must do it alone.

'Be still, and know that God is here.' And I knew he was, but I was afraid. Afraid of asking a girl sixteen years younger than myself to share the future with me; afraid of my crippled back and legs and my diseased heart; afraid of the memory of Clare living with me in reproach. It was dark and very silent when I left the chapel and walked through the sleeping house to my room: and I was still afraid.

I took her to Barnstaple the following morning and saw her off on the train to London. We were quiet, hating the moment of departure, both of us now fearful we were letting the future slip out of our grasp. She leant out of the window, forcing herself to remain calm. 'Will I see you again?' she asked quietly.

'Yes! Yes, of course. Look, I'm spending the weekend with my sister in Sussex, then a week in Kent before going back to the Retreat House. What time do you knock off from work?'

'Five.'

'I'll meet you at the coach station at Victoria at 5.30 on Tuesday. That's a promise!' The train started moving and in a panic I walked after it: 'Jo, don't forget the Doone Valley—it was real—Johanna . . . .'

I saw her lips moving in reply but the train and the noise carried her and the words away. Conscious only that I was making a mess of things I walked slowly back to my car. With her face vividly before me I drove up onto the moors, but the moors gave me no comfort that day. Back at the house I collected my gear and made preparations to leave early the next morning, and by eight-thirty on the Saturday I was once more part of a crawling mass of traffic slowly trickling out of the West Country.

Somehow the weekend passed. As the hours ticked by the dreamlike quality of the world in which I was moving grew, and still I could not make up my mind what I should, or should not say to Johanna on the following Tuesday. Round and round in my head chased the twin problems: had I, a physical crock, the moral right to ask a girl years younger than myself to marry me. And what about Clare? Where, in all this, did Clare fit in? On the Monday I returned to stay with an aunt in the village in Kent, to the very cottage where Clare and I had lived together for so many years before we moved up to the Midlands. My confusion grew as I wandered round the old familiar scenes and saw the well-remembered and well-loved faces. In the village church I tried to find the solution; but there was only stillness, and the knowledge that this was something which I must work out alone in my own heart.

Mentally exhausted I went to bed early and fell into a deep sleep, to be woken abruptly hours later—by what? Maybe only by the workings of an over-laden imagination. Maybe by a dream. Maybe by the wind that whispered over that hill-top in Kent. But maybe by a laugh—a rich, throaty laugh which I had known for seventeen years: an expression of gaiety, of humour, and of reassurance. I do not know—will not know while I remain in this mortality. All I can know is that on the very edge of awareness I was touched by—intelligence? Being? A keen, cool counter-awareness of self? I do not know, only that as I felt complete relaxation stealing over me I heard the voice in the darkness of the night, or my mind: 'Such a clot, Jim. Stop running away—it's all right. It's all all right!'

And the vision of a bright future opened up.

Outside Victoria coach station at the height of the rush hour is the devil of a time and place in which to propose to anybody. A million tired feet hurried by, the reek and fume of London going home to its tea and television assaulting the nostrils, the roar of a hundred thousand damn-you-Jack vehicles battered the ear-drums. I saw her turn the corner and scan the parked cars, an expression half fearful, half expectant on her face; watched the sun come out as I scrambled out of my seat and started forward to meet her

The great city around us vanished as we stood together in an isolation as old as mankind himself.

'Jim, you're here!'

'Yes, it's been a horrible weekend.'

'Horrible!'

'Johanna—darling, will you marry me?'

She laughed, the sound snatched away by the passing thunder, the curious grins of passers-by unheeded: 'You bet I will!' she said.

3

RUMBLINGS

SUCH was the girl who became my second wife. The girl who blossomed into a woman, became the mother of our two children, and, during this past year, has lived and coped with the imminence of death. My death.

Certainly that February night in 1971 when my overworked heart at last decided to go on strike, both Johanna and I came face to face with death. For me it was a simple question of telling death to get lost, and then surviving. But for Johanna it was the end of a six years' tightrope, and the beginning of month upon month of living upon one thing only: faith.

I came through that heart attack, and twenty-four hours later was planning a return to work. A month later I was still in bed, shaken in my belief that my damaged heart would do what I told it to, and weighed down under a blanket of exhaustion I seemed incapable of throwing off. Not for thirty years had I known such weakness, and I did not take kindly to it. My doctor came to see me regularly, brooded over my chest, told Johanna emphatically to keep me absolutely quiet, and departed muttering about second opinions. Much of the time I slept; all of the while acutely aware that the stalwart organ inside my chest had changed into a different gear, and was making very heavy weather at the slighest demand put upon it.

Three people came into the picture during that month: friends who were to become deeply involved in the events towards which we were unknowingly headed. Pat and Christopher lived in Bristol, where he was the rector of the city churches. Tim was also a priest, rector of the unspoilt village of Sapperton, near Cirencester. Like Johanna and myself, all three believed in the power of a compassionate God to heal and make whole; indeed, acting as a channel for divine healing was a large part of Tim's ministry, and he travelled the country extensively bringing comfort to many who suffered in body, mind or spirit.

Now they came to see me together, and, first of many times in the following months, they prayed with Johanna for my healing. What form that healing might take not one of us had any idea; but as the weeks went by, despite the fact that I remained hard pushed by my protesting heart, all of us became convinced that healed I would be. We knew the doctor was afraid I might have another heart attack at any time, yet persistently the thought grew in each of us that I was not yet destined to bow out of this mortal sphere of life.

The doctor was certainly concerned by my condition, and made an appointment for me to see a consultant physician at the local hospital in Leamington. On April the first a friend drove me to the hospital: there followed the usual interminable wait which seems to be an integral part of all out-patients departments, anywhere, then I was being quizzed by the doctor who was to trigger off the most explosive event in my not uneventful life. He knew from that first moment where my heart was heading and how it might be possible to deal with it. Not that he spilled many beans during that first meeting! He said that my heart was in a very bad condition—that I knew probably better than anyone—but he could not give any prognosis, or advice, until he had more information on me. I would have to be X-rayed, blood tests taken, and would I please come and see him again in one weeks' time?

Muttering about long-winded doctors, I rejoined my friend and was driven home. Next morning I was duly X-rayed and relieved of a large syringe-full of blood, and settled down to wait for my next appointment with the consultant. My heart remained tiresome and my temper not at its sweetest.

I will not forget that second visit to the consultant in a hurry. Once again he examined me minutely, studied X-rays and pathology reports in heavy silence, then at last sat down and started talking. His opening shot hit the target.

'I want you in hospital,' he said, 'right away.'

'*In* hospital! What the blazes for?'

He sighed, leaning forward over his desk. 'Mr Ross, I don't have to pretend to you about the condition of your heart—you've known yourself that it's been seriously diseased for years; and you also know that during these last few weeks it's taken a bit of a nose-dive. Right?'

'Yes, right. In the past it always used to recover fairly quickly after letting me down. This time it hasn't.'

'No. And there are two reasons. First, I think your heart has an infection in it: sort of nests of bugs collected in those bad valves of yours. The blood tests and my own observations indicate bacterial endocarditis and . . .'

'Bacterial? Is that the same thing they called infective endocarditis when I had it thirty years ago?'

'Yes.'

'But—for the love of mike! I was flat-out last time. So ill I didn't know what was happening for weeks. I'm not like that now!'

'No. You had it very severely when you were a boy, with complications as well I should think, now you appear to have a mild infection. But infection all the same, and I can only find out definitely whether you have got it, and treat it, in hospital.'

I digested this in silence. Then: 'Damnation take the thing! Why the heck has it gone bad on me suddenly like this? And how long will all this take?'

'Mr Ross, don't abuse your heart now', said the consultant mildly. 'You know as well as I do that thirty years is an incredible length of time for valves in the state yours are in to have kept going—and kept you going reasonably well, especially when on your own admission you've pushed them to the limit. No, the question, rather, is how they have managed to keep going for so long! Now, I want you in hospital right away. The sooner you're admitted, the sooner we shall know where we are.'

'What do you mean—right away?'

'Now.'

'Sorry, I'm going home and explaining this lot to my wife. I'll come in tomorrow—as apparently I must', I ended rebelliously.

'I can't force you, but you should. Ten o'clock?'

'Twelve. My wife will have a certain amount to sort out. Couple of hours can't make much difference.'

He cocked a tolerant eye at me. 'You're an obstinate man, Mr Ross. Still, it's a trait which will probably come in useful.'

'How long will I be in, Doctor?'

'A week or ten days to do a series of blood-culture tests on you, and get the results. If they are negative, home you go. Positive, and it will be six weeks in hospital having penicillin jabs in your rump at regular intervals. O.K.?'

It had to be. I had no alternative. But what an infernal nuisance it all was. Johanna and the children would be badly upset by this out-of-the-blue shock. Six weeks! I turned back to the consultant who was watching me closely.

'I'm certain I haven't got endocarditis', I said firmly. 'My heart's tired, that's all. Once it's recovered from that attack . . .'

'Mr Ross, there might be repeats. It's not just a matter of endocarditis, you realise.'

I frowned at him. 'What do you mean?'

'I mean your valves. The mitral and aortic. They're in bad shape, you know.'

'They have been for years.'

'But there comes a time when bad becomes worse. And when worse has got to be dealt with—if that's possible. It's not wise to let you have many more attacks like your recent one if we can prevent them.'

I was still staring at him, not the faintest idea of what he was getting at. He gazed back, his eyes summing-up, searching. Then . . .

'Mr Ross, have you ever thought there might come a time when your heart could benefit from surgery?'

I must have looked half-witted. 'What sort of surgery?' I demanded at length. 'Years ago—Oh Lord, fifteen years ago at least I asked if there wasn't some surgical way of strengthening my heart, and all the specialists said no. What do you mean?'

'I mean,' he answered carefully, 'that it is perfectly possible these days to replace diseased heart valves with artificial ones. You must know that, though.'

'I've heard of it.' Who hadn't? Experiments using pig's valves to replace human one's. Plastic valve replacement—yes, I'd read about it in magazines and papers. Generally it was written up in a sensational fashion, and to the accompaniment of whole columns of print defending or attacking the practice. Replacement surgery, they called it, and it apparently engendered as much heat as did heart-transplants to the people who disliked this whole branch of experimental medicine. Oh yes, I'd heard of it. But—on me? I had never even dreamt of such a thing. Why should I when my heart had managed to keep jogging along over the years?

'Well, it's just a thought', said the consultant briskly. 'First we've got to check whether you have got endocarditis, and deal with it if necessary. Then, if you agree, I'd like you to see a cardiologist and get his opinion. I suggest we take one step at a time. Now, go home and sort things out and I'll see you in the ward tomorrow.'

For ten frustrating days I occupied a bed in that Leamington hospital, while blood was regularly removed from my arms and sent to the path lab for culturing. They needed eight clear cultures running to pronounce me not a victim of bacterial endocarditis. My hopes rose as the first seven were as clear as a whistle: number eight was positive. I swore briefly when the young house-man cheerfully gave me the results: 'Now what?' I demanded.

'Now we start again and do another series. One positive: it's not positive enough if you see what I mean. Either way.'

I glared at him. 'Look, my blood is OK, I've been feeling better ever since I came in here. Let's just accept that everything is settling down nicely, and send me home. Right?'

'Wrong. Anyway, we've got to decide on the next step. I'll grant you seem a lot better in your general health, but you've still got a couple of right grotty valves inside you. Remember?'

I wasn't likely to forget. Ever since my talk with the consultant, Johanna and I had been only too conscious of my valves. Both she and the children had been upset at my abrupt departure into hospital, but she had bounced back quickly and on the surface appeared quite unruffled. Now, during her daily visits to me, we discussed lightheartedly the possibility that I might have to have an operation on my heart at some time, but admitted that our knowledge of what exactly that would entail was nil. Vaguely we both began to be aware that we were caught up in something which could prove far bigger than either of us had ever dreamed, but we refused to be pessimistic about the future, looking instead at the fact that I was at last feeling better, and drawing out of the exhaustion which had followed my heart attack.

It was good to feel some strength returning to my body, and as the days went by, I began to tell myself that the whole thing was probably one of those false alarms doctors sometimes delight in. My blood would prove all right, and as for my valves—well, they had coped for enough years now in all consequence, and they could darned well go on coping. Surgery? Maybe in the remote future, but there was no sense in even thinking about it yet. All right. I knew my heart had taken a hammering in the past couple of months, and maybe death was trying to put in a take-over bid on my body: but I could still cope. And intended to go on coping.

And while I had to sit it out in hospital, life wasn't all that bad. The hospital building was old and far too cramped to serve a growing town like Leamington: true. But the ward was cheerful, the nurses and junior doctors efficient and friendly, the blood-suckers who daily attacked my arms equally so, and my fellow-patients were variegated enough to make life interesting. Best of all, I was not confined to bed, and as I grew stronger I began to wander about at will.

After more than a quarter of a century free from hospitals I had forgotten just how pithy they can be. Two incidents (out of several) reminded me of this fact, and did much to restore my jaded sense of humour. Granted, they were pretty earthy, but one needs a spot of earthiness when death will persist in peering over one's shoulder. Anyway, I do.

One of the patients was well known to me, a man I had met in Coventry some years before, and whom I knew to possess a ripe sense of humour. He was an intellectual, and had little time for foolishness either in himself or others. And all of us in our ward were subjected to a considerable degree of foolishness from one of our fellow-patients. This was a man who, to put things mildly, was a bit mixed up.

Half his time he spent trying to evangelise us, lecturing us by the hour on the love of God, sin, salvation and repentance. The rest of the time he spent in attacking coloured people: a practice which pushed up the tempers of most of us—being cared for with skill and compassion by a staff of nurses more than fifty per cent of whom were coloured did not exactly endear us to the opinions of our potted Enoch Powell.

However, we held our peace until the night of The Supper. Without being too rude to that hospital, the standard of its food was not precisely that of the Ritz. What exactly they did to it none of us was ever able to make out, but the meals which came up three times a day were more—intriguing, shall I say, than *Cordon Bleu*. And The Supper was a corker.

My next-door neighbour, Jeff, had ordered minced chicken. He took one look at it, swallowed, then asked in hollow tones:

'Tide gone out or something? What is it—no, don't answer, keep the conversation clean.'

David, my Coventry friend, had been so misguided as to order a rissole. He also uncovered his plate, blenched, and backed hastily away. 'What have you got?' he asked me faintly.

I had hit the jackpot. On my menu sheet the previous day I had ticked off some sort of diced ham and rice risotto. Now I wished I had not been so bold. The other patients boggled at the alarming offering on my plate. 'Maybe it's meant to be good for my valves', I said weakly.

Our evangelistic-colour-conscious friend decided it was time for reproof.

' 'Ere,' he rumbled, 'You didn't orta grumble about the food like wot you do.'—Pregnant pause—'The Lord give you that food, 'E did.'

David leaned forward across his offending supper with an indescribable expression on his face:

'Then the Lord can bloody well have it back again!' he hooted.

I don't think my own collapse would have been quite so acute had I not caught sight of our comfortable, placid sister standing in the doorway with tears of sheer bliss running down her cheeks. Like the man said—we gave it back.

Then there was my little encounter with—Bridie, I think I'll call her. Not her correct name, but one which suits her and her Irish blood well enough. Bridie was a ward orderly: a cheerful, bouncing woman in her forties who didn't know what it meant to come into the ward without a smile on her face, and some improbable—and generally appallingly vulgar—story on her tongue. She had an unerring instinct for picking out patients who felt low, and propping them up with her own unquenchable spirits. She made a beeline for me the day I learned I would have to have a second series of blood cultures taken. I was wandering down the ward towards the loo, feeling distinctly unsociable, when she loomed up in front of me.

'Seen me bruises?' she hissed in a conspiratorial whisper.

'No, have you hurt . . .'

Before I could finish my question, or even move out of range, she lifted her skirt high up to display a huge, blackened bruise on her ample thigh. Feebly I stared at the generous, battered limb.

'Good grief, how did you do that?' I blurted out.

'Ah, dear God, me husband it was—rampaging, lusty great stallion.' She nodded at me profoundly: 'Give it to me, he did, becos I didn't get me drawers off quick enough last night . . .' She came up closer to me, dark eyes twinkling with merriment—'Hey, boyo, if ye're going out to the sluice would ye like to see what else the . . .'

'Bridie, belt up!' I fled, cannoned into someone, and realised that once again our ubiquitous sister had not missed a syllable. She steadied me, murmured something about my blood pressure, and courteously stood aside to let me pass. What she said to Bridie I don't know, but I got the impression that our shrewd sister did not believe in leaning too hard on her walking bottle of tonic.

The second series of tests was negative, so, reluctantly, the consultant decided to give me the benefit of the doubt and let me return home. He was curiously loathe to release me, and right up to the last moment when I was dressed and waiting with the friend who was to drive me home, he kept me on tenterhooks by refusing to come out with a direct yes or no. He had insisted on seeing me once more before I left, and I sat in the ward seething with impatience, and quite determined that once through the doors I was finished with hospitals. For good!

He arrived at last with his retinue of house-men and sisters, and cocked an eye at me over his spectacles.

'You're sure you're not conning me?' he asked.

'What the . . . what do you mean "Conning you"?'

'You really do feel better? You're not just saying so to get home?'

'I really do feel a lot better! Why on earth should I—con you, as you put it?'

'Hum. And you're not so tired?'

'Oh, I'm tired, but nothing like I was for the first month after that attack. Doctor, I am clear on this endocarditis thing, aren't I?'

'I should say so—yes, yes, I think you're clear.'

'Well then?'

He muttered something, searched through my notes, and once again eyed me up and down as though I was some sort of unusual specimen.

'Well—you can go home. But I want you to promise me

you will do absolutely nothing. You're to rest and go on resting, and I'll make an appointment for you to see a consultant cardiologist who examines outpatients at the Warwick Hospital. And as soon as possible. Agreed?'

'OK Doctor—You're worried about me having another attack, aren't you?'

'I'm worried about your valves.' He moved restlessly, then grabbed my wrist, fingers probing for my pulse. 'Frankly, I've never known anyone with valves in the state yours are in just walk into hospital—and then walk out again. They really are in a very poor condition, and if you do have another attack it will take you very much longer to get over it. Assuming you do get over it', he ended quietly.

'I see.' So the endocarditis scare was almost a detail. 'OK, I'll be careful.'

'Please do. I'll confess I'd much rather keep you in hospital right under my eye until the cardiologist examines you, but I suppose if I suggested it you'd walk out on me.'

'I'm afraid I would.'

'Then go home—and, I repeat, rest! Get as strong and fit as you can, but please don't overdo it. If the cardiologist does recommend an operation—and I believe he will—he will want you as fit as possible before it's done. You realise that open-heart surgery on a comparatively fit person entails far less risk than when performed on a patient in a state of failure?'

'I'm beginning to think I'm coming up against the same sort of choice that confronted Mr Hobson', I remarked, far more lightly than I felt.

'One step at a time. Now, get off home, and don't forget—no exertion!'

'Where is it all heading?' asked Johanna later that same day.

'I think to an operation', I replied slowly. 'His chief worry seems to be whether I'll even get that far.'

'Because you've got a time-bomb in your chest.' It was a statement, not a query. 'Darling, don't you think we'd better cancel our holiday now?'

'No!' Once again we had booked to go back to the mountains and valleys of Wales which we both loved so much. After the last few months of frustration and weakness I did not feel like foregoing it now, especially when I could feel strength returning to my body. 'No, let's get away and forget my bally heart for a while. Even if the cardiologist does recommend an op, I expect it will take months before they do it. Isn't there a waiting list for most operations these days?'

'Yes, but . . .' She looked at me curiously, 'I don't think you will have to wait long if they decide to operate. Which is odd when you consider that a fortnight ago neither of us had ever dreamed of an op. What do you feel about it, Jim—an operation of that magnitude, I mean?'

'Not much.'

Which could well rank as one of the under-statements of the year.

When I saw him in mid-May the cardiologist was forthright, and cautious. Forthright about the state of my heart, cautious over talking about an operation before I had undergone heart catheterisation and been thoroughly examined by a cardiac surgeon.

'The last word must lie with the surgeon', he said. 'He will operate only if he feels he has a reasonable chance of success, and he'll need the results of the catheterisation and rather a lot of other tests as well, I'm afraid, before he'll commit himself. We're in something of a dilemma which we want to sort out. I think we're going to find that replacement of those worn-out valves of yours is the only chance you have of any reasonable expectancy of life. But certain things have to be done before we make the final decision—and meantime it's vital you don't impose any added strain on your heart.'

'Then you agree with the consultant that future prospects with my heart as it is are less than rosy?'

'I know he has been completely honest with you, and I intend to be also. Your future prospects are extremely limited. Your mitral and aortic valves are leaking badly and under great strain. As is the rest of the heart muscle, which can only take so much extra burden before it—stops. That might not happen tomorrow, or even next week; but six months, a year, possibly even two years if you are very careful, and I think your heart would be unable to function.' He shook his head at me gently: 'Thirty years is a very long time for those valves to have kept going, Mr Ross.'

'That's what the consultant said; seems I was right about Mr Hobson', I murmured absently.

'I beg your pardon?'

'Hobson, the bloke with the grotty choice. Doctor, this op—what would it entail?'

'It's impossible to say yet, but replacement of both those valves is my belief.'

'With plastic ones?'

'Well—with artificial ones. You'll find out all the details when we get to that stage.'

'And obviously there's some sort of risk attached to an op like this. How big a risk?'

'Twenty per cent, maybe thirty-three and a third per cent risk of failure in your case.' He looked at me intently. 'You realise you're not a straightforward case, Mr Ross?'

'Why not? I'm skinny, I've got a good constitution, I don't smoke—haven't done so for over five years. I'd have thought I was a darned good case. What's the problem?'

There was quite a pause, and I watched the cardiologist and his house-man exchanging glances. Then he nodded at me. 'You've got ankylosing spondylitis of the spine, osteo-arthritis of your right hip, and hardening of the bone structure of your ribs due to years of arthritis. These things present problems, but—look, let's leave all this to the surgeon. They're his province, and it's not worth even discussing these things until after the catheterisation and his own examination of you. How soon can you come into hospital for me to do the catheterisation? I'll want you in for about ten days.'

So I had got another spell in hospital before me. And another if they decided to do the operation. If! With the option a short period of heart attacks until the fatal one they could alter that if to when! And to blazes with my bones and problems and risks.

'Which hospital?' I asked, 'Here or Leamington?'

'Neither. The cardiac unit for this area is at the Walsgrave Hospital in Coventry. You know—the new one, it's only been open about a year.'

'I've heard of it. Don't local people call it the Coventry Hilton?'

He grinned. 'Yes, and it's very modern. Certainly the heart unit is as up to date as you'll find anywhere, and everything we need for doing our tests on you is there.'

'And the op?'

'Depends entirely on the surgeon. He might want you to go to the Queen Elizabeth Hospital in Birmingham.'

'Why?'

'Well, they're very experienced over there.'

'And they're not at the Walsgrave?'

'Good heavens, of course they are! The unit may be new, but the thoracic-cardiac team has built up fourteen years experience at Hertford Hill here in Warwick. They moved to Coventry when the new unit was opened at the Walsgrave.'

'Then let's count the Q.E. out—far too complicated for

my wife to have me over there. I'll take the Walsgrave.'

'For the tests, yes', said the cardiologist firmly. 'As far as any operation is concerned, let's leave that to the surgeon. I repeat, there are considerable complications in your case. Now, when can you come in? The sooner we start the better.'

I looked moodily at the young house-man who was quietly watching his superior at work. Truth to tell I didn't want to go in at all. I felt I was being rushed along by circumstances which were too big, too demanding, and over which I had next to no control. Damn, damn my heart for letting me down now! A wife and children I loved, all the work as a free-lance that I needed (and where the deuce would those precious contracts be after this lot?), and now everything was confused and in jeopardy. But—there was the real rub: what all these doctors were really saying was that my life was in acute jeopardy. Tell them to take their catheterisations and operations and get lost—and the future shrank to a little time of heart failure, growing weakness, and death. Accept their offer of surgery—not that it had yet been offered—and the future was still a narrowing path which might, or might not, lead to a future with Johanna and the children. You pays your money and you takes your choice. Johanna and the children: I had no choice.

'I understand you'll want me fit if I'm to have this operation', I said at length. 'I'm booked to go away to Wales on holiday during June, and I'd like to go. Partly for my family's sake, and partly because it will give me a chance to get really fit. As fit as my wretched valves will let me, that is. What about doing the catheterisation lark in July?'

'I'd rather do it next week.'

'And I'd rather it waited until after I've had a holiday', I said stubbornly. Was I just putting it off? I've often wondered since. While I could say next month or after a holiday—in the future, any time but now, things like heart catheters and open-heart surgery remained remote and academic. Something which might happen at some point, some time. But not yet. I don't think I had still grasped quite how acute the choices were.

'Very well, but make it a holiday. Do you like the mountains?'

'Very much. I'm jolly good at crawling up Cader.'

'Well, no climbing this time! You're to rest and relax and treat your heart to a little consideration for a change. Positively no climbing! How do you feel?'

'Better than I've done for months.'

'That's probably a pity! But, seriously, I want you to get as fit as possible during these next few weeks. I don't want us to have to deal with you in a state of failure.'

'Doctor, I'll be as placid as a contented cow.'

A suspicious eye followed me out of his consulting-room.

'That I doubt', he remarked dryly.

4

HOBSON'S CHOICE

We lay on the warm sand and idly watched the children playing at the water's edge.

'I think I'll write a book about all this', I remarked sleepily.

Johanna turned over to get the other side cooked. 'I thought you would.'

'And I might as well start now while it's all happening.'

'But, darling, we don't even know yet if you'll have the op. Supposing . . .'

'Suppose nothing. I'm going to both start and finish the book: right?'

'Right.' But we both knew what she was thinking. I looked down at my near-naked body, deeply tanned, the thrust of my heart easily visible on the smooth, unscarred chest. Impossible to believe that this was real. That I was sprawling on a sun-lit beach feeling strong and well, while in a matter of a few weeks or months that same chest might be split open and the heart inside it—my heart—cut open. Yet that was probably the reality, and Johanna was already feeling the pain of it even if I wasn't. For me 'the operation' was still an academic possibility, something stored away in the future, and I could not get bothered about something which had not yet happened. But Jo had admitted to me the night before that sometimes she looked at me enjoying myself with the children on the beach, in the sea or up in the hills, and a wave of hurt would almost overwhelm her as a vision of how desperately ill I could become before the end of the year swamped her senses. Intuitively she knew that each hour, each day, we walked closer to a razor's edge, and she clung onto the one anchor she knew would not let us down in a sea of insecurity: her faith. It was a faith we shared.

Faith is a suspect word nowadays. If you use it you're immediately on trial as an old-hat religionist, out of tune with modern theological thought, out of touch with modern science and technology—and man's ability to be very much the master of his own destiny. Faith to many people, both the man in the street and all too many men in clerical collars, is little more than a foolish persistence in blindly trusting in a supernatural being—a God—outside oneself, one's experience, outside and apart from the universe which 'man come of age' has the power to know and control. Faith, for many moderns, smacks of clinging to a 'god' of our own making; trusting in a fable invented by non-scientific man to help him in a frightening, suffering world he did not understand; of turning in desperation to a fairy-godfather paternalistic-Santa-Claus figure when the problems of living got too big for him. Faith has become out of step with mankind who has grown up to become the godhead of his own twentieth-century technology. It is effete, irrelevant, totally superfluous.

But, when you look hard at our modern world the technological grin of triumph tends to become a grimace. The lordship of science is seen to be all too often a tyranny. Man come of age appears more like an adolescent frantically seeking for something which constantly eludes him. Man may have found that he does not need a God to explain the things which once puzzled and frightened him; he may not need to appeal to his tribal medicine-man—Christian or pagan—to alleviate his sufferings; he may be confident in his own ability to control his own environment, his own problems, his own fate, but he remains strangely troubled and uncertain in his new-found lordship. He has forgotten, or tried to dismiss, what man has acknowledged in the million-odd years he has been a man. That there is an 'Other' outside ourselves, who is also infinitely more real and enduring than ourselves. And that the Other is so closely interwoven into the living fabric of mankind, that to ignore him is to suffer self-mutilation. An amputation of an essential part of our very being.

I believe in God: the creator in whom I live and who lives in me. If I did not, the whole fabric of this muddled world would become a nonsense. The more the science and technology of mankind throws new light on the hidden corners of the universe, the more the immensity of our non-knowing becomes revealed, and the more the existence of something other than man—something we call God—becomes evident.

I have not always believed in God, still less in the being and meaning of Christ. For considerably more than half my life the former was only a myth, the latter a sop for the credulous. But it was the world of science which started turning my hard-held views upside-down: it was through an amateur's interest in and study of the heavens that I first advanced from agnosticism to a stage where, when the crunch came, I was able to accept the Christian God of love. All my life the heavens have fascinated me—the remoteness of the stars, the mystery of the beginnings of the universe, the silent wanderings of the solar planets through space.

How unimaginably tiny man seemed to all that! How insignificant the self-styled lords of creation appeared when set against their background of the universe! A handful of sentient creatures struggling and squabbling on the surface of an insignificant planet orbiting a minor star at the periphery of a galaxy the proportions of which made one's brain reel. And beyond that galaxy—itself only modest in size by astronomical standards—more galaxies, and more. More to the very limits of belief: certainly to the limits of the devices which men had invented to probe the ocean of space around him. Put him against this background and man became puny, a detail in the cosmos—and yet it was at this point that the real stature and glory of the existence of mankind became apparent.

When I look up at the stars on a clear and silent night I know in every part of my being that all this vastness was created—had to be created to make any sense or logic at all. Through the study of the stars man's knowledge of the evolution of the universe is being pushed to the limits of space and time, and as he probes deeper into space so further pieces of the creative puzzle seem to fall into place. Hoyle's theory of Continuous State, or the 'Big Bang'—you may take your choice, either seem to conform with the fragments of truth steadily coming within the grasp of man's knowledge.

Almost we are back at the beginning. Either there was an almighty bang from which all matter, galaxies, stars, planets, you and me—everything began once and for all, or matter and therefore the universe is constantly being created: no beginning, no middle, no end. It just is. But still the question is left begging: what went before? The Big Bang did not explode from nothing. Continuous State does not create from nothing. One is ultimately brought sharp up against the unavoidable question: what was or happened before *that*? Why did that happen? Where, before there ever was a Big Bang or a Continuous State, did the circumstances come from which arose these creative acts? What triggered it all off? What caused it to *be*?

Irresistibly I find that, in the last analysis, I am brought up against one thing only: mind. Intelligence. A creator.

A creator far more worthy of man's respect than the hoary and largely 'big brother' creator who has dominated Western Christianity for centuries. A creator who, even in the simple

Genesis story, is revealed as intelligence capable of forming the stars—intelligence, that is the key word! God is love and life and light—yes, if you believe in him at all he is all these things. But, over and above, he is intelligence itself, from which everything within the ken of man flows.

Including healing. And by healing I mean that which comes through the doctors' drugs and the surgeons' knife quite as much as that which can come quietly, and without human intervention, directly from the power and compassion of God.

'Healing' is another of those suspect words. There are members of various religious sects who condemn and reject all medical or surgical treatment, all resource to drugs and the skills of men. They are wrong! And there are those, the majority of people in this modern western world it would appear, who scoff at or dismiss as absurd any idea that 'God' can heal solely by some mysterious power of his own. And they, too, are wrong! The God who is in us equally as we are in him, who is at the root and core of our whole being as well as being the Other, so almighty that he is almost beyond our limited comprehension: that God uses every channel of healing open to him. Because wholeness, of which physical healing is only a part, is the primary will of God for all mankind; and if we do not achieve wholeness we do not have to search far for the reasons why.

As Christians, Johanna and I find the answers to the why and how of wholeness in Christ. In his life, his teaching, his death, and in his continued living. On that last, like millions of Christians before us, we are prepared to stake everything. And the Christ in whom we believe told people to pray, taught them how to pray, prayed himself. Painstakingly, over the years, I have learnt how to pray, to communicate with God, and although I shall never be very much good at it I have found that it enables me to face the humdrum of life, the good and the bad, the joys and the sorrows, with a peace of mind I never even knew existed before I became a Christian.

So, as individuals, together, with one or two close friends, Johanna and I prayed about the situation which now confronted us: the Hobson's choice in which death seemed to hold far too many of the best cards. By praying I do not mean we battered God with pleas to pull his finger out and immediately transform my diseased heart valves into healthy ones: that sort of thing, in my view, is not prayer. Instead we sought to find out what we should do in this tricky situation—what was the right thing to do. What our response should be to every new problem presented to us in a fluid and unpredictable situation.

I think it was St Ignatius who once told his companions 'to pray as if everything depended on God, and to act as if everything depended on oneself'. A little thought reveals just how profound that comment was. In a way prayer is the deliberate affirmation that we are prepared, under the guidance of God, to do all we can to find the right solutions to our human problems; and if that means we are seeking healing, to explore all possible human means available to us as part of our trusting in God's wish for us to find wholeness. We should pray for healing if we believe in a compassionate God—yes, of course we should. But part of that prayer should be that we may be led to avail ourselves, seriously and to the best of our ability, of all the techniques of modern medical science which man has so painstakingly built up. And having asked God for guidance, one should then leave the problem confidently with him, knowing that guidance will come. To keep nagging God for reassurance is profitable to no one.

It was this attitude to God and prayer which enabled Johanna and myself to relax on holiday without constantly being plagued by my heart. Johanna admitted to having her bad moments, and there were times when I was well aware that the pump in my chest was working strictly under protest. Breathlessness was my constant companion, especially at night, palpitations continued acutely enough to make me wonder at times just what the blazes was going on inside me, and pain which could hit from my breastbone to finger-tips was never very far away.

Nevertheless, during those two sunlit weeks in Wales my heart generally took a back seat, and we enjoyed ourselves. On the whole I obeyed the strictures of the cardiologist and kept my feet off the flanks of those green and enticing mountains. Only once did I fall from grace and follow the two children, Jonathan and Rebecca, to the summit of an insignificant peak a few miles north of Cader Idris. And standing on the top, with my valves flapping and breath scattered to the wind—standing looking far out over the hills and valleys, the lakes and the green loveliness which is Wales, I knew with a deep and absolute conviction that I would be back. Not merely that summer, as we were already planning, but next year, and other years in a future which was still completely hidden.

Hobson's choice? I watched the children running down the hill below me: two wind-blown bits of humanity running into a future which I intended to share with them. 'Pray as if everything depended on God, and act as if everything depended on oneself!' I followed them down the hill and into that unknown future.

Two days after returning home I was admitted to the Walsgrave Hospital in Coventry for the catheterisation tests. I cannot pretend I was looking forward to this—having tubes threaded along my viens and thence into the heart itself did not exactly strike me as a pleasurable entertainment. Still, it was a necessary part of intensive cardiac investigation nowadays, so the sooner it was done the sooner I would know what the score was.

I had heard and read a good deal about the Walsgrave Hospital during the year since it had been officially opened by the Queen in 1970, but I had not yet seen it, let alone been inside. I knew it was ultra-modern, that local people referred to it as the Coventry Hilton, and that it worked on what was known as the 'progressive nursing' technique. I did not know what the latter meant, had heard it criticised in some quarters, and was prepared to dislike it on the principle that I had learned all there was to learn about hospitals thirty years ago, thank you very much, and did not approve of fooling about with well-tried methods.

Not for the first time in my life I discovered that I can be rather too hasty in my pre-judgements.

The same friend who had taken me to the Leamington hospital, Lewis, drove Jo and myself to the hospital ('It's becoming a habit', he remarked), and as we swung off the main road and the hospital came into full view we all three gaped like country cousins up in the big city for the first time. It was indeed modern.

The hospital complex is built—building, rather, because it is not yet finished—on the very outskirts of Coventry. It looks out over the great industrial sprawl which is modern Coventry, but backs onto countryside which is (as yet) virtually unspoilt. The main building consists of four great, connected wings built on rising ground, flanked by the separate blocks (architecturally splendid or deplorable: it depends on your taste) of the nurses' home, doctors' residence, maternity hospital, and all the mass of technical and administrative buildings which a great modern hospital demands. Standing on its own green acres, the whole complex is uncrowded, roomy and easy on the eye: a far cry from the ancient, huddled buildings I had become used to under the heading of 'hospitals' during my lifetime.

Still gaping we walked into Reception.

'Do you think we've made a mistake and come to an airport?' murmured Lewis.

'Let's ask for your flight number and see what happens', suggested Jo.

I said nothing. It's too big, too modern, I was thinking. It will be as impersonal as a computer and I'll be nothing but a case number to be processed by a lot of automatons who may be clinically efficient but will be about as human as Dr Who's Daleks. Damnation take my heart for letting me in for this lot!

I knew I was wrong even as the girl at the reception desk checked my details and clipped a plastic nametag round my wrist. She was the reverse of impersonal, as was the woman who escorted me up to the pre-operative section of the thoracic unit: Ward C3. Everywhere was spacious: reception area, corridors, lifts, the hub at the junction of the four wings where the lift disgorged us—and the ward itself. First impressions slunk hurriedly away as we were greeted by a cheerful staff-nurse, and led down a wide corridor lined with one, two or four-bed rooms on one side, and by an impressive array of bathrooms, lavatories, sluices, kitchens, treatment and store rooms on the other. Halfway down, the corridor widened out into what was called the 'nurses station'—the administrative centre of the ward—and then we were being shown into a room containing four beds, three men, and a splendid view out over the city of Coventry. Everything gleamed with light paint, stainless steel and aluminium fittings, silent floors, long glass panels looking out onto the corridor, and built-in fittings which revealed that scrimping on finances had certainly not been in the minds of the planners of this magnificent hospital.

But further surprises were to come. Even as I was being shown my bed, locker, and cupboard for my clothes to hang in (ye gods—in a hospital!), and we were still gawping like country cousins, I realised that women, girls and children—none of them nurses—kept passing up and down the corridor outside. A dark-haired woman in her forties grinned cheerfully and waved through the corridor window as she passed: I turned to the staff-nurse. 'Do you mean to say you actually mix the sexes here?' I queried.

'Oh yes. Good for the staff and patients. Rooms like this are for the same sex, of course, but that's only common sense. Otherwise it's a men, women and children ward—and the parents of children when necessary. You're all hearts and lungs so you're all in one unit together. Sensible, and good for the morale of patients, incidentally.'

She introduced us to the three other men in the room, all dressed and all looking remarkably carefree. There was no need to get into bed, I discovered, in fact patients were expected to dress each day unless obviously too ill to do so. C3 was the ward from which tests, exploratory examinations and investigations were conducted, and there was no point in flopping about in bed unless one had to. Still feeling slightly dazed, I said goodbye to Johanna and Lewis and settled into my new and comfortable surroundings.

From that first moment I was enormously impressed by (and grateful for) something it is often difficult to achieve in the average large ward in an orthodox hospital where constant comings and goings by staff and patients are unavoidable: peace and quietness. I have been in wards in the past where, during the day, the resemblance to Piccadilly was too close for comfort, and, by night, the cacophony of restless, sick, and all too frequently windy patients, staff, and outside noises of people and traffic make sleep virtually impossible. In this purpose-built hospital there was little to disturb a calm which seemed to cover the whole place. Maybe the staff had their community upheavals and turmoils—I do not doubt it. But for the average patient there was quietness, peace, and a sense of everything working with great efficiency but little fuss for his or her well-being.

Even the food was good! Unless a patient was confined to bed, everyone had their meals together in a pleasant dining/common room, where the mingling of the sexes was civilised and stimulating. There were no rigid rules about lights-out, or settling to sleep at too early an hour—and on C3 at least, where most patients were fit enough to bath and attend to their own hygiene, we were not woken up at the appallingly early hour most hospitals still adhere to. Early morning tea was laid on around seven o'clock, breakfast at eight, and, unless one was booked for some test or other, the day would jog through on peacefully oiled wheels. A quick check with the ward sister or staff-nurse on duty to ensure I wasn't wanted by some doctor, by path or the X-ray department, and I was free to wander at will through this hospital with a difference. On what was called the Lower Ground Floor was a bank, a shop, a coffee bar—all set in a large roomy area with dozens of comfortable seats where patients and visitors could relax and feel completely free from a 'hospital atmosphere'. All these amenities were run by the Friends of Walsgrave Hospital, a body of some four hundred men and women from local parishes who did an incredible amount of voluntary work in the hospital. Not only was the shop and bar on Lower Ground Floor run by voluntary help, but drinks trolleys which came round the wards each morning and evening, the care and layout of flowers, the very comprehensive library, the mobile shop which came to every ward each day—all were run by this small army of volunteers who regularly gave up a great deal of their spare time in which to do this work. Even more, I was regularly visited by members of the Church of England Mens' Society, who came to sit and talk and help pass the time; they were also quite prepared to, and often did turn their hands to helping with patients on the wards in a dozen different ways when the chronic shortage of staff from which all hospitals suffer put in an extra squeeze. It is impossible to estimate just how much work this company of volunteers did, but it is absolutely certain that without them the hospital would either have had to struggle to find more permanent nursing and ward-orderly staff, or fairly drastically curtail its activities. No praise is too high for those people who give their time and help to such hospitals as the Walsgrave—the evidence that ordinary people in ordinary communities care for their fellow men and women is overwhelmingly strong.

Six floors up I discovered the chapels (opposite the ladys' hairdressing salon!) : one large enough to take a congregation of—at a guess—a couple of hundred, and used by both Anglicans and non-conformists; and a small one for the use of Roman Catholic priests, staff and patients. Both were beautifully designed and appointed, and both had offices adjoining them for the use of the chaplains. On my very first day in the hospital the resident Anglican Chaplain came to see me, and I was impressed to learn that he knew not only my name but a great deal about my medical history. He had been medically briefed before he came to see me, and as time went by I was to find out that the co-operation between consultants and the Chaplain was a close and workaday relationship. Here, the Chaplain was not an optional extra for patients needing some sort of spiritual comfort—he was a member of the team.

I think I heard that word 'team' more than most others during my time in the thoracic unit of the Walsgrave Hospital. It was rammed into me right from the start, even before I had the catheterisation; teamwork was the foundation on which the whole unit was built. It embraced surgeons, doctors, the technician who runs the 'pump' (heart-lung machine), sisters, nurses, X-ray technicians, pathology technicians, physiotherapists—the patient himself, and the Chaplain. Here was medicine honed to the sharpest edge: a pooling of skills and knowledge which worked with extraordinary efficiency towards a desired end. Before three more months were out I was to know at first hand just how close-knit and effective was that team.

For five days I led the quiet life, interrupted only by examinations from various doctors, generous blood-lettings, X-rays and the testing of copious quantities of my urine. Then came the catheterisation performed by the cardiologist, followed by a rather tense wait for the results. Apart from a sore arm I had no ill-effects—none had been expected, and my heart continued to remain more or less peaceful. Three days before we would have the results of the catheterisation, the cardiologist had said, and I spent much of them wandering round the hospital with fellow-patients, drinking interminable cups of coffee at the bar on the Lower Ground Floor, and wondering if it was worth breaking out to a pub temptingly sited only a couple of hundred yards from the hospital. Johanna visited regularly—no restrictions on visiting here—the days ticked quietly by, and the moment I had been impatiently half-dreading arrived.

I felt my pulse beat faster as the cardiologist entered the ward with his house-man and the sister, and curtains were drawn around my bed. He nodded, smiling, and once again went over my chest with his stethoscope.

'Where do we stand?' I asked flatly.

'You badly need an operation for replacement of your mitral and aortic valves, and I advise you to have it as soon as we can arrange it—though, you understand, the last word still rests with the cardiac surgeon.'

'And you think the rest of the heart will be able to stand the op?'

'The catheterisation readings on the other chambers of your heart were reasonable. The whole muscle is grossly swollen, of course, but—yes, there's a good chance it can cope.' He hesitated, then: 'I can't guarantee the surgeon will undertake the operation. You see, there are other complications—your bent spine and that very rigid rib structure. These could present problems.'

'But . . . Doctor, do the results of the catheterisation confirm that without the operation my heart is virtually finished? I prefer to know exactly where I stand.'

He sat down on the bed, looking at me very directly. 'And of course you must. We wouldn't dream of advising you to have this operation, or attempting it without you being absolutely clear on what your condition is now—and its prospects—and what chances such an operation might hold out. You'll find if you do have the operation you will be briefed on it, and its aftermath, down to the last detail.' He smiled, 'You're a member of a team, you know, and we must have your full co-operation.'

'But my heart as it is?' I persisted, 'It's got no future, has it?'

'Very little, I'm afraid. Both those diseased valves are leaking badly and have calcified almost into uselessness. You need new valves, Mr Ross, and I strongly advise you to have them—providing the surgeon agrees. I'm afraid at the moment it can only be one step at a time. You will have to wait to see the surgeon. I'd have liked you to have stayed in hospital and seen him tomorrow, but I had forgotten he was due to leave on holiday this week. He won't be back until the second week in August, but I'll make an appointment for you to see him at Warwick directly he returns.'

Oh my God, more delays! Just how long would this stop-go business drag on? Not that this was anybody's fault. Surgeons, like other people and more than many, needed their holidays, and I would just have to wait. But there was a nasty sinking feeling inside me I had to try and get resolved now.

'Doctor, surely the operation can be done—or at least attempted. Why should my ribs and spine matter all that much?'

'Because they are rigid, and the whole technical problem of getting to your heart could be made very much more difficult than is normal. Your neck, also, is badly set as you know. But let's not worry about all that at the moment. We'll assume that the operation is feasible, and you will see the surgeon in August. If he agrees an operation is necessary—will you consent to it?'

I looked down at my chest, at the always-visible, uneven thrust beside the left nipple, at the dark tan I had collected in Wales only a couple of weeks earlier. Should I agree to such an operation, which seemed to get more risky and more complicated every time it was mentioned? After all, I was feeling pretty fit again, and this wasn't the first time my heart had been on the blink during the thirty years trek from its first collapse. Could I not trust my own tough constitution and the faith I had always put in my diseased heart to cope—and go on coping? Thirty years ago top-rate doctors had not expected me to live: yet I had lived! Shouldn't that be sufficient for me to trust in my own recuperative powers again? Wouldn't it be wiser just to forget all about any operation? Was it fair to Johanna and the children to have an operation which, apparently, I might not even survive? Although, equally, was it fair to them not to attempt the operation when the alternative was being spelt out to me in words of two syllables by top-rank consultants?

What did I really think about it? What, *what* was the right thing to do? To operate or not to operate, that is the question, I thought confusedly—Oh, hells bells, of course there can't be any doubt! I don't need catheterisations and tests to tell me that this thing inside me is packing up! Not after the last thirty years of knowing every mood of it. It's done its stint with those fantastically tough valves; it's had a good go but now I can feel with every beat that it's refusing to work any more overtime. Yes, I'm feeling pretty well, but if I'm to be really honest I have to admit I have already gone off the peak of well-being I attained only a few weeks ago. The thing is sliding; that wretched exhaustion is waiting not far off in the background; when the next attack comes, will there be enough strength in reserve to fight it?

'Well?' asked the cardiologist, 'Will you have the operation—if it is offered?'

'Yes, providing my wife agrees. She must have a say in the decision. After all, she'll have the tougher part in this business—whether I have the op or not.'

'The surgeon won't operate unless he is assured your wife is one hundred per cent with you. And he will want to interview her himself. All right, you can go on home, but once again . . .'

'Do nothing: I know! What does nothing mean? We are thinking of going back to Wales again for another week: my young son is booked to have his tonsils out at the end of August and it will build him up. Any objections to me buzzing off to the mountains again?'

'I can't very well stop you. But you know what I mean: nothing, positively nothing strenuous. When are you going?'

'Middle of August.'

'Then you'll see the surgeon before you go.' He turned and opened the curtains to leave me: 'You're not worried?'

'No. I'll be glad when I know where I stand over the op—that's all. Thank you for being so frank.'

'Goodbye for now. Good luck.'

Pat and Chris came up from Bristol, and Tim from Sapperton, to discuss and pray about the situation, and give me the laying on of hands. The Bishop of Coventry, Dr Cuthbert Bardsley, a friend of long standing, was drawn closer into the circle of those intent on my healing. He had been to see me regularly since my collapse in February; now his support as the tension began to rise was invaluable. Nora, a Coventry friend, started an intense period of prayer which was to culminate in a non-stop vigil at a time when I, at least, was incapable of any prayer. And from family, friends and strangers alike, both locally and from all over the country, assurances of their thoughts and prayers began to increase from a stream to a flood. A second team was being built up—or was it part of the same one?—which was to play a part none of us could really calculate when we reached the crunch.

But as July ended and the cold, wet beginning of that August of 1971 began to pass, none of us yet knew what the crunch was to be. The pump in my body strove to keep going; 'the operation' still remained something unreal, pushed away in an unknowable future; death still jogged along beside us, an unseen but ever-present companion who might yet play his trump.

And on a day of showers and sunshine I went to see the cardiac surgeon.

5

DECISIONS

Jo came flying out to the car when I got back from Warwick.

'Well?' she demanded, 'Is he going to do it?'

'It's a bit complicated.' In the kitchen I routed out a bottle of beer and tried to get my thoughts into some sort of order.

'It can't be much more complicated than it's been up to now! Darling, you don't mean he won't do it?'

'Not exactly. It's just—well, he's wondering if the Walsgrave team, including himself, have got the experience to tackle someone with my blasted crooked spine and rigid rib structure. Oh, I know the cardiologist warned us my bones might cause difficulties, but I didn't expect this.' I drew a deep breath and faced Jo squarely: 'This surgeon is wondering if it wouldn't be better to send me down to the National Heart Hospital in London. And even then he isn't sure whether they would undertake to do it.'

Jo sat down slowly on a stool, dismay all over her face. 'London!' she exclaimed.

'Yes. But—I told him I darned well don't want to go to London! Oh, I know it's a marvellous hospital there, but—I *liked* this chap, and I've got a strong feeling he should be the one to do it.'

'What was he like?'

'Big. Quiet. Didn't say very much. But if a man who we know is a first-class heart surgeon says he isn't sure whether he's got the experience to do an op like this on a peculiar carcase like mine—well, dammit, it shows he's got humility, and only big people possess that trait!' I slammed my glass down on the table emphatically: 'I don't want anyone else to do the job!'

'But suppose he insists on London?'

'Then I'll insist on the Walsgrave. It's my heart, after all.'

'Oh Lord, this does complicate things, doesn't it? Where do we go from here?'

'He wants me in hospital again. As soon after Johnny has had his tonsils out as possible—around the end of the month. I told him it would be impossible for you if Jonathan and I were in different hospitals, in different towns both at the same time, and he said he would see everything was fixed smoothly. He wants me for about a week to do a lot more tests . . .'

'What, more?'

'Yep. He said he wants me in to turn his team loose on me—doctors, anaesthetists, physiotherapy bods, nursing team, path lab: the lot. Then when they have all reported their findings to him he'll make up his mind. And not before. Apparently my stiff neck is quite a considerable snag—bigger even than my ribs, maybe, but that's a problem for the anaesthetist.'

'But—why?'

'Well, at some stage they've got to shove a dirty great tube down inside it, and that could be awkward. Though he did say they could probably overcome that by doing a tracheotomy.'

'You mean making a hole in your throat?'

'Yes.'

'Charming! This gets better and better. Darling, did he say anything about the risks?'

I swirled the beer round in my glass, gazing into the golden whirlpool. But there was no way to soften this one, and Jo wouldn't want me to.

'I'm afraid the odds have lengthened, love. What with my

spine and ribs—not to mention the heart itself—he thinks it could be as high as a fifty per cent chance of failure. Maybe higher. That's why he's thinking about London.'

'Fifty per cent!' She drew a deep breath and I could see the shock in her eyes. 'All right, but without the operation the chances are non-existent. Did he confirm that?'

'Yes. Both these valves are finished, and it's only a matter of time—and a pretty short time at that—before the rest of the heart packs up altogether under the strain.'

'So you'll have the op?'

'Of course—as long as you agree.'

'And, darling, if he insists on London you'll go, won't you? Oh, I know it will be terribly inconvenient . . .'

'Grief, it will be more than that! It makes it impossible for you. How the dickens can you look after the children when they will need you more than ever before in their lives, and come down to visit me in London? And what about the actual time of the operation? You'll want to be either at or near the hospital—how do we work all that lot out?'

'Leave it, Jim! If we have to work it out we will. We're not exactly without friends. But, darling . . .' She swung round sharply as a memory struck her: 'You said something about maybe even London wouldn't be willing to do the operation—does that mean the surgeon really believes it can't be done at all? By anybody?'

'It's a possibility—and we have been warned before, you know. The risks might be too great.'

'But they've got to do it! Someone has *got* to—they can't just let you fade out! It doesn't matter what the risk is, at least it's worth trying. I don't think I can bear the thought of seeing you have another and maybe another heart attack, just getting weaker all the time until you die! And it would be terrible for the children. At least with the operation there must be some hope.'

'There is, Jo, don't let's worry about that side of it—I'm darned sure either London or the Walsgrave will be able to do it. Someone must have operated on a heart case with peculiar bones before, and if they haven't it's high time someone had a go! God knows, diseased valves and arthritis aren't all that unusual. And, maybe I'm just imagining things, but I've got a strong feeling it's going to be the surgeon I saw this morning.' I hesitated, trying to sort out what I did mean. 'I don't know why, but I'm certain he's the man for the job. I only saw him for a few minutes but I'd trust him literally with—well, with my life.'

There was a long silence, each of us busy with our own thoughts.

'Jim, it's an awfully big risk', said Jo at last. And she almost succeeded in keeping the pain out of her voice. 'What do you feel about that side of it all?'

I wandered to the window and looked out. In bright sunshine, the rain-clouds temporarily chased far away, Rebecca was trotting up and down the garden pushing Bear in her wobbly pushchair. Every time she rounded a corner Bear fell out, to be picked up, roundly scolded, and thrust back onto his precarious perch again. She was talking non-stop, oblivious to everything but the reality of her private world of sun and grass and Bear.

Jo came up beside me and put her arm round my waist. 'What are you thinking about?' she asked quietly.

I grinned at her. 'Winnie-the-Pooh', I replied.

'Pooh? What on earth do you mean?'

Again Bear fell out of the pushchair. Rebecca picked him up, spoke to him severely, and set off down the garden. 'Winnie-the-Pooh,' I said, 'has a philosophy I've subscribed to since I was Rebecca's age. Do you remember that story in *The House at Pooh Corner*? The one where Owl's house is blown down in a gale? Pooh and Piglet are walking through the Hundred Acre Wood, and Piglet is getting rather nervous as he listens to the wind roaring through the treetops above him. Eventually, when he's getting very worried, he says: "Supposing a tree fell down, Pooh, when we were underneath it?"

'And Pooh gives this a lot of thought, and at last he says: "Supposing it didn't!" '

The little figure in the garden suddenly glanced towards the house, saw us and waved. Bear promptly fell out of the pushchair. Equally promptly he was picked up, scolded, and put back again. What on earth did risks matter when the stakes were as high as that?

'OK,' said Jo, 'Supposing it didn't!'

So we went back to the cottage in Wales for another week. And again, after weeks of bad weather, the sun smiled on us as we wandered in the mountains or lazed by the sea. My heart behaved itself, more or less, although it was becoming obvious to both of us that it was heading towards more trouble. Breathlessness, which had been a problem for years, was now so acute that even a reasonable night's sleep had become a rarity. Tiredness and pain, again old companions, were now rather too obtrusive for comfort. My arthritic bones were awkward and unco-operative, probably due to enforced inactivity. Always in the past I had coped with my osteoarthritis by making the joints work. My theory that a seized-up hip could damned well unseize itself by walking up a steep hill or standing on a ladder painting the house may not always have had finesse, but it had worked for a very long time. Now, in the months since my heart had become temperamental, my physical activity had got so limited that arthritic joints and rheumatic muscles had stiffened, movement was difficult, and this in turn appeared to be laying its own strain on the heart. It had been at its worst in May when I first started getting about again after weeks in bed and my first stay in hospital (the 'month of the hip in the year of the heart', as we named it), and although by August I was somewhat less creaky, walking still held its tiresome moments—as my heart was not slow to inform me. Many times I remembered that if it had not been for my heart giving out on me, I might now be walking on a brand-new plastic or steel hip-joint—with all the advantages this would bestow on other bent and bony systems in my frame—and I vowed that directly I was well and truly recovered from the heart operation (when, not if), I would start nagging the doctors for that new hip.

'What are you trying to do?' asked Jo, 'get a reduction for bulk-buying? Why not have a hair-piece while you're about it, and get really groovy?'

'Because I don't need a hair-piece, thank you,' I replied loftily, 'I'm extremely well-off for hair.'

'If you mean your beard, I'm pretty sure they'll insist it comes off before operating on you.'

Once again we were on the beach, watching the children darting about in the sand and sea. I almost fell off my beach-chair at Jo's monstrous suggestion.

'Take my beard off: like stink they will! Why—why, good grief, that's not a boy's beard of two whiskers and a bit of dandruff: that's a beard! All twenty-two years growth of it. Regularly pruned and treated with the best compost. Dammit, they're going to operate on my heart, not my tonsils! I refuse, absolutely refuse point-blank to have any doctor, nurse or sacriligious barber touch a hair of it! Why, I'll . . . I'll . . .' Words failed me and I lay back limply, stroking the threatened fungus tenderly.

'You'll what?' asked Jo mercilessly.

'I think I'll go for a dip with Johnny', I replied evasively, and retired with dignity down the beach.

I suppose it was partly obstinacy which made me go in the sea every day, even though more than once I only just had the strength to crawl out and wait for Jo to help me back to our chairs. But the sea and sun were warm, the eyes of the cardiologist a long way away, and the years-old determination not to let my life be ruled by heart and arthritis was far too strong to be completely thrust aside now. It would have been so easy all those years ago to have accepted the status of 'invalid', to have let a floundering heart and permanent lameness dictate the pace of my life. Far easier than constantly prodding the unwilling horse to keep going. But I do not like being dictated to, be the dictator a person or my own body. Such an attitude has probably made me do many foolish things in my life, but it has added a dimension to living which has made the stars shine brighter and the grass grow greener. For more than a quarter of a century prudence has tried to suggest that I cosset my heart and bones, but I believe if I had listened too much to prudence I would have turned either into a chronic invalid, or been dead a long time ago. So I fooled in the sea with Jonathan, walked in the hills, and sat outside a near-by hotel with Jo, watching the children exploring the grounds while we knocked back some well-earned sustenance. On Sunday we went to church in our Welsh village, and became part of a congregation praising God as the Welsh have done for uncounted generations. And the pump in my chest, faltering and uncertain, managed to keep going.

The light-hearted days in the sun ran out and we turned our backs on Wales to trek back to the Midlands, and more spells in hospital. Not that I set the pace this time: this one was Jonathan's affair. With remarkable aplomb for a five-year-old he packed a case with all the things he considered necessary for a tonsillectomy (toilet articles and pyjamas being noticeably lacking among his effects), and was ready two hours before his parents to leave for the hospital in Leamington.

Five days later, minus tonsils, he was home again, viewing with considerable superiority the fact that his father also might have to undergo an operation. After all he, Jonathan, had already had his operation, and he was completely assured that all other operations should pass off with the same ease. The blessing of this piece of childish logic in the months to come could not be over-rated.

At the end of the first week of September I re-entered the Walsgrave Hospital for the complex series of tests which would determine whether or not I was a suitable candidate for having my mitral and aortic valves replaced with artificial ones. Once again I found myself in ward C3, with copious quantities of blood being removed from me; yet more X-rays taken and added to the by now splendid picture gallery of my insides which the hospital had accumulated; twenty-four hour collections of urine being whisked away to the path lab for detailed chemical analysis; my lungs examined for capacity, strength and general efficiency; unbelievable yards of electro-cardiogram traces clicked off and bundled away like so many paper streamers for earnest contemplation by the surgeon and cardiologist; and, although I did not realise it immediately, a close psychological watch kept on me to ascertain if I had a reasonable level of mental and spiritual equipment to help me cope with the massive type of open-heart surgery envisaged.

The consultant anaesthetist of the heart unit, a splendid type of doctor with an extraordinarily penetrating mind, plus both his assistants—two very attractive young women—examined me, shook their heads over my beard and prophesied cheerfully that *that* would have to come off, but declared they could otherwise manage. True, they might have to perform a tracheotomy on me, but that decision could wait until I was laid out on the operating table. Physiotherapy bounced on my chest, announced sternly that I had not breathed properly for at least twenty years, and proceeded to teach me how to perform this basic function.

Feeling slightly battered, I asked the ward sister to fill me out somewhat on what the operation actually entailed.

'You'll be briefed before they do it—if they do it,' she said, 'So there's no need for me to go into many details now. What sort of things do you want to know?'

'Well—where will the surgeon make his incision, for a start: north to south, east to west, or a mixture of both?'

'North to south, from the base of your neck straight down the breastbone to about—Oh, let me see, about an inch north of your navel.'

'And how do they fasten the breastbone together again: glue?'

'Clips. Metal ones which will be a permanent part of your anatomy for the rest of your life. OK, next question.'

'The heart-lung machine: how long will I be on that during the op? In other words, how long will a machine keep me alive while my heart is out of action?'

'The by-pass, we call it, or just the pump. It depends on the duration of the operation. In your case it will take a good six hours, which means you'll be on the by-pass—Oh, I expect about two to three hours.'

'And after I come round, what about my lungs? How do they take to being flattened for a few hours?'

'When you come round you'll be breathing through a special sort of respirator—a ventilator which will actually do your breathing for you. As you come off that so physiotherapy will help you use your lungs properly again, hence the importance of all the exercises your physiotherapist, Miss Kay, has asked you to do now.'

'It sounds like a pleasant party game! What sort of anaesthetic do they use?'

'You'll have to ask the anaesthetist, because that's rather complicated. But they will introduce a strong relaxant into the anaesthetic which may, or may not, get your neck back sufficiently for them to dispense with a tracheotomy. They use curare.'

'You mean the hoary old South American Indians' poison? You're kidding!'

'I am not. Curare is widely used in thoracic surgery: it's a very powerful relaxing agent.'

'So the Indians obviously thought when they pumped their enemies full of it. What else have you got on the agenda?'

'Plenty, but it can wait for your briefing. By the way, the surgeon will be coming in on Saturday morning, and he wants to see you. He'll let you know whether he's prepared to operate then', she finished evenly.

'Hold on—what about this shaving lark? Will I really have to lose my beard?'

'I'm afraid so, plus a lot more. Lung cases are only shaved down to the middle, but cardiac jobs are shaved from the face to the toes: north, south, east and west!'

'Oh Lord, I'll look like a chicken ready for the oven! Sister, no one is to touch my face with a razor after the op, then by the time I leave hospital maybe I'll look human again. OK?'

'It's a deal—I'll pass it on to A3.' Of course, I was forgetting. My present ward, C3, was pre-operative. I would be prepared for surgery here, and go to theatre from here, but I would wake up in the super-intensive-care unit on A3. This was what progressive nursing was all about. Now I had begun to know more about it I could see the arguments both for and against. One school of thought felt very strongly that the sisters and nurses who had to care for a patient after a serious operation should be the ones to prepare and pre-med him. Thus they would know their patient in advance, and he or she would recover consciousness after an operation to recognise familiar faces tending them. The argument had points in its favour, but there was another side, one which, as a patient, I was to come to appreciate more keenly. The run-down towards an operation on C3 was peaceful and unhurried; one was comparatively well among other patients who were also comparatively well: the affect of this atmosphere on morale was powerful. If a patient should be admitted, prepared, and taken to theatre straight from A3 (as had to happen sometimes in emergencies) then, comparatively well, that patient would be prepared among other patients going through all the trauma of major post-operative surgery.

The pros and cons of these two methods were debated many times during my weeks as a patient in the Walsgrave Hospital, but in the end I came down firmly on the side of progressive nursing. I can understand that many nurses would prefer to have their patients from the moment they are admitted to hospital until the time they leave, well on the road to recovery—there must be enormous satisfaction in seeing both the beginning and end of a case. But from the point of view of a patient, and one who had to contend with what the surgeon once described to me as a 'maximus' operation, I believe that the advantages of progressive nursing far outweigh the disadvantages. The concentration of sheer skill extended by teams dealing exclusively with one period of a patient's progress has to be experienced to be really understood.

Saturday, September the eleventh, and I walked down the ward to see the surgeon in his consultant's room at the entrance to A3. I cannot pretend I did not feel tense: so much depended on what was said now. Yes, he would operate? No, he would not? London? The team did not believe anyone could operate? My pulse was not at its steadiest when I opened the door and went in.

He eyed me keenly as I sat down. 'All right, Mr Ross, I'm prepared to give it a go if you are. There are difficulties but my team believes we can overcome them. What do you say?'

I shrugged, aware of little but immense relief that a concrete decision had been made. 'Thank you—yes, I'll have it. I don't see that I've got a great deal of choice.'

'It's not easy, I'll grant you, but both the choice and the decision have to be yours,' he said quietly, 'I can only advise.'

'When would you like to do it?'

'As soon as possible. I'm losing my registrar soon and I would like to get you in before he leaves. I don't want to have to wait until I've found and trained a new man—that would mean the beginning of next year, and that could be too long with your heart in the condition it is now in. Now, can you phone your wife and get her to come in and see me? I want to talk to her as well as you.'

'Yes, surely, when . . .'

'Now.'

An hour later we both sat facing the cardiac surgeon.

'I've agreed to operate on your husband, Mrs Ross, and he's willing to go ahead. Let's say we both look upon it as a challenge. Now—what are your feelings?'

I looked closely at Jo, aware that the surgeon was searching her with his eyes. Her cheeks were rather flushed, her eyes bright, but she was completely composed.

'Is it really a matter of Hobson's choice?' she asked.

'Yes. There's very little future for your husband with his valves in their present state. I'm afraid they are finished. Operating is the one real chance we have.'

'Well—thank God for that. It would have been pretty hard to take if you had said no, you couldn't operate at all. And you'll do it yourself, here at the Walsgrave?'

'Yes.'

She smiled at me: 'That's another relief; we won't have to work out complicated travelling arrangements. When will it be?'

He explained, and added, 'Now, ask any questions you like.'

'How long will the operation take?'

'Well,' the surgeon smiled, 'If I'm at my peak and my team are at their peak—six hours.'

'You will be at your peak!' stated Jo firmly. 'What happens at the time of the operation—about me, I mean? Do you want me here at the hospital, or do you prefer me not hanging about like an expectant father?'

'I'd like you to stay at home until I phone you. I know it will seem a very long day, and be extremely difficult for you to wait patiently, but I promise to phone the moment it's over. And I'd like you to make arrangements so that you can stay here at the hospital for the night. There's a room on the ward where you will be quite comfortable, and I'd like you to be on the spot. Will you do that?'

'Of course. I expect to have a friend with me—is that all right?'

'Yes, there are two divan beds in the room.' He paused a moment: 'You do both appreciate that the risks involved are —considerable?'

'Fifty-fifty if we're lucky', answered Jo quietly. 'Yes, we know that. But, what is the biggest risk—in the whole thing, I mean? I'd like to know.'

'Let's just say that the entire operation entails risk, but assuming we all get through the operation OK, one of the diciest moments for your husband will be when he comes off the ventilator afterwards. You know? When the lungs have to start earning their own living again. But the biggest problem is mine, a technical one: the mechanics of getting to your husband's heart . . .'

'You mean his stiff ribs?'

'Yes. That and the spine. The neck—they all present problems, but I believe we can overcome them.'

'How long will Jim be in hospital—after the operation, I mean?'

'Don't pin me down, but—Oh, a month. It's a pretty traumatic affair, you know. Anything else?'

'Yes. When it's all over and Jim is back home, will you come and knock off a bottle of champagne with us to celebrate?'

A slow smile spread across the surgeon's face. 'I'd be delighted to', he said.

6

COUNTDOWN

I RETURNED home to await the letter recalling me to hospital for the operation. It was an unreal interlude.

The surgeon had said 'as soon as possible', but what that actually meant we did not know: it could mean weeks or days. We hoped it would be the latter. Although we both had complete confidence in the outcome of the operation, it was inevitable that we should feel a steady screwing up of tension as each day passed by. For, despite our confidence, both of us had moments when the realisation hit us at full strength that we could be living the last short part of our life together. This knowledge did not depress us, neither did it make us morbid—they were happy days when we were more vividly aware of ourselves, our love and our children than ever before. We cleared the decks for action: we made sure our Wills were in order, that correspondence was up to date, no bills were left outstanding, the car was in good condition and odd jobs about the house were dealt with. And we told the children that I would soon have to go back into hospital again. It had been a difficult year for them and Rebecca, at least, was showing signs that her sense of security was being somewhat knocked about as her father kept disappearing into hospital. But as far as possible we had to try to be honest with them: to treat them only as children and not as people would have been a betrayal. My initial collapse in February had meant a collapse of one part of their world. Without any warning the father they had always known as active and energetic suddenly became someone sick in bed or in hospital; a father who, even when up and about, was no longer able to romp and play with them as he had done for as long as they could remember. It had meant a radical readjustment for them, and the news that I would soon have to go back to hospital was a hefty pill to swallow.

'How long for?' demanded Jonathan, and being told about six weeks he was reduced to uttering in tones of great disgust his favourite swear-word: 'Schweppes!' But they had been forewarned, and any shocks the next few weeks might bring would not fall on unprepared ground. Whatever the outcome of the operation Jo was going to have to carry a heavy burden for a considerable time, and maintaining a steady, secure home-life for the children would not be the least of her problems.

One strange piece of defence mechanism in both of us still placed the operation in the future: no date had yet been set, therefore the whole thing was still a remote and somewhat academic exercise—it wasn't yet actually with us, and while it remained remote it also remained unreal. The surgeon had told us that one week's hospital preparation was usually needed before valve replacement surgery, but in my case, because of my arthritic condition, he would probably want two weeks. Even this crumb of knowledge helped to keep in the future the operation we wanted over and done with. We were both affected by the same dichotomy: part of us wanted the operation tomorrow, while part of us would have liked to have been able to put it off for ever.

'I feel like that song', said Jo to me once: 'You know—"Stop the world, I want to get off!" '

But the world does not stop merely because one wants it to, so instead we made our plans to cope with the world as it was. And that involved, more than anything or anybody else, our friend Pat from Bristol.

Pat is a woman of rare quality, although she would be forthright in denying any such thing. Like all that small band of people who possess deep spiritual faith and strength, she has her feet solidly on the ground—common sense is a hallmark of those who walk close to God. She epitomises the best in modern women: competent, intelligent, extremely attractive, independent and, important to Jo in the coming weeks, she is an excellent driver. For a long time we had known that Jo should have someone with her at the time of the operation, someone who shared our faith and could be relied upon to 'keep their cool' during an emergency. Pat, with her three children away at boarding school, had said she could come; now we phoned her and clinched it. Whenever the operation occurred, she would be with Jo twenty-four hours in advance. I felt a deep sense of relief at the knowledge that when the countdown on this particular venture was over, Jo would not be alone.

During these days we came to experience something which Jo was to know even more vividly in the weeks and months ahead. The term 'the caring community' has become something of a cliché in modern sociological and Church circles; the aim of social workers and many local authorities is to foster a 'caring community'—which basically, I suppose, means encouraging people to recognise that each one of us is his brother's keeper. One facet of this caring community began to show up strongly as the days of waiting went by; a facet which, despite the stresses and strains in modern society, I believe to be widespread. Any number of our neighbours in the parish, close friends or complete strangers, went out of their way to let us know that they were concerned for us, our family, and the adventure which now faced us. People Jo scarcely or never knew would stop her when she was out shopping, to tell her they would be thinking of us or praying for us: indeed, it is remarkable, in this apparently Godless age, just how many people do not hesitate to assure someone within their community who has hit an emergency that they will pray for them. And my experience leads me to believe that in the great majority of cases this is no trite sop, but utterly sincere. Permissive and violent our modern society may be; but the average, ordinary man or woman does care about other ordinary men and women. I have heard it said many times that modern man has become hopelessly selfish, turned in on himself, complacent or apathetic about the problems and needs of his neighbour—whether that neighbour lives next door or out in the Third World. And I do not believe it. Of course complacency and apathy exist: they always have and I suspect they always will, but in very much larger measure exists at least the wish to help, even if, as is so often the case, it seems virtually impossible to do anything practical oneself.

Jo and I, particularly Jo, met this desire to help unmistakably and movingly. A desire of ordinary people to let us know they were solidly behind us. That we were not alone. That they cared a great deal about the outcome of the next few weeks. And it should be added that the community in which Jo and I live is very much a suburban community, where people are commonly supposed to live their own lives, mind their own business, and surround themselves with a shell of self-interest. Maybe some do: more do not. Our society is richer in compassion than the way-out fringe, the detractors, the noisy marxists, maoists and anarchists would have us believe.

Six days after my return home from the Walsgrave Hospital, the letter arrived. It was Friday, September seventeenth, a beautiful, sunny day, the beginning of that perfect autumn weather which was to continue week after week until late November. Jo watched me slowly as I opened the letter: both of us knew what it contained, and both of us felt the same sinking sensation.

'When do they want you?' asked Jo quietly.

'Next Tuesday, the twenty-first.'

'Four days.' She drew a deep breath. 'Then if they take a fortnight to prepare you that will mean the operation about —on October the fifth.'

'I should think so.' I took her hands in mine and for a long moment we gazed at one another. 'It's an odd feeling, isn't it?'

'Yes. We've expected it, and waited to know, and it's all been pretty tense-making, but now it's come as a shock. When shall we tell the children?'

'Wait until Monday, then we'll tell them—without trimmings—that I've got to go into hospital for an operation. Johnny is well clued up on operations now—he'll be OK. And Becca . . .' I shook my head, 'I don't know. You'll just have to give them both an extra dollop of love, Jo, while I'm away.'

'Do you want me to bring them in to see you before the op? Just at the weekend, I mean. Or will that be too difficult for you? We'll both have to be frightfully matter-of-fact about it if I do.'

'Bring them in.' The future was rushing down on us, turning into the Now with remorseless speed. 'It will help to have seen them when things get a bit ropey.' I squeezed her hands hard—'I am going to survive this op, you know Jo.'

Her hands returned my pressure. 'I know you are!' she stated firmly.

Saying goodbye to the children meant playing it very cool indeed. Anything else would have been intolerable.

'Goodbye, Johnno—don't forget you're the man of the house again. Help Mummy look after Becca.'

'Um. 'Bye Daddy.' He looked at me sternly for a few moments, school cap askew, dark eyes unwavering. Then: 'Six weeks—Schweppes!' And he was gone, running off to school with the supreme confidence which knew that my tatty valves would be winkled out as quickly and efficiently as his own tonsils had been removed.

Damn that emotion which rises up in the throat to choke; the thoughts and fears which swirl through the brain and are far better left alone. Goodbye Jonathan: for six weeks? Or for this lifetime?

'Cheerio, Becca. Daddy's got to go back to hospital again —you remember? The operation?'

'Becca come to hospital too. 'Ave mine tonsils out.'

'Not right now, love.' A quick kiss—'You'll be good?'

'Yes. You come back soon?'

The problems are very serious, Mr. Ross. You must understand that in your case the risk of failure might be more than fifty per cent. To hell with it: supposing the tree doesn't fall down!

'Yes, soon! Enjoy yourself at play school.'

Driving the nine miles to the hospital in a state of total unreality; the Warwickshire countryside, the familiar streets of Coventry slipping past in a dream. Saying goodbye to Jo, and our vicar who had driven us in, and watching her walk with quick feet and high head back to the car—'S'long, Jo. I'll phone when I get the date of the op. But that's bound to be another fortnight yet.'

But it wasn't. 'You're booked for next Tuesday', said the ward sister on C3 when I asked her. 'The registrar is leaving on October the second, and the surgeon has been very anxious to get you in before he goes. You start the pre-op tests right now.'

So it was only one week away. With a slam the future and the surmising over the date of the 'maximus' operation were gone. Reality rushed in: one week—six days, rather, before the whole of the world as Johanna and I knew it changed drastically in one way or another.

Was I afraid? On the whole I thought not. This was a

different feeling to fear: more a come-on-for-God's-sake-get-on-with-it anticipation. Now I knew how a parachutist felt in the last seconds before jumping from his burning plane, or an astronaut must feel as he sits on the top of his multi-thousand ton bomb waiting for the blast-off. The weeks and months of tension and waiting were gone; now all must be clinical, controlled working with this remarkable medical team towards one end only: life.

For me, even the time for prayer had almost gone. Now I must rely on that other team—the close-knit circle of family and friends surrounding Jo, and the hundreds of people all over the country whose prayers were solidly with us. And even as I sat in my sunlit room on C3 I became aware of a great calm descending on me, a sense of peace greater than I have ever known before. Whatever happened to me in one week's time, this affair was *right.*

I watched Jo as she came into the hospital that evening. 'Next Tuesday!' she had exclaimed when I phoned her, 'Only a week.' And then—'Oh, I'm glad!' Now she walked into the Lower Ground Floor where I was waiting for her, dressed in flaming red slacks, a trendy blouse which caused most male heads in range to swing round in admiration at her figure (a man has to be very ill indeed not to notice a woman's vital statistics), and a tranquillity on her face which was quite unassumed.

Whoever it was who first called women the weaker sex (certainly a man) must have been out of his tiny mind. They have a toughness, a durability which few men possess. Okay, I was the one in hospital and the heart plumbing had to be performed on me. But Jo had the infinitely harder task of waiting. Waiting through the countdown. Waiting through the interminable silent hours of the operation itself. Waiting with all senses screwed to a peak of awareness; with two small children to look after to whom she must try not to communicate emotion or fears. Waiting, when the chips were really down, to discover if she was still a wife, or a widow.

'Hi! What's the score?'

'It's all go. Doctors, physio-bods, dolly-birds rushing up asking me to pee all the time, and path syphoning off so much blood I've been put on Guinness to offset acute anaemia. It's the routine as last time—only more so! And I won't be able to see you down here after tomorrow.'

'Why not? It makes a break to have coffee here.'

'Strict orders. I'm confined to barracks from Thursday morning. Partly to get me as quiet and placid as possible by next Tuesday, partly to avoid catching anything. For the love of mike don't get a cold—if I caught one they would probably cancel the op. And that would be a bit too much. Did you ring Pat?'

'Yes, she'll be with me by Monday afternoon at the latest, and she's just going to stay until—until we know where we are.'

'Thank God for that. Jo, I've been finding out quite a lot more about the operation, chiefly from my physiotherapist. This afternoon when she was assaulting me she said: "You can ask as many questions as you like now, and we'll give you the answers. The more briefed you are the better. But after the operation we want you to do exactly what you're told, and not waste time or breath on questions." I gather that I'll feel as though I've had an argument with a double-decker bus for about a week following the op. The registrar confirmed that—darling, you realise I'm going to look a bit of a shambles when I come round from the anaesthetic?'

'I've realised that for weeks', she replied. 'But—did you learn anything else?'

'Yes. Replacement valves made of plastic do exist, but I won't be getting them.'

'Then what are they made of—you don't mean they're going to try giving you animal valves?'

'Not at all: metal ones. They are the latest medical marvel invented by some genius in the United States, who seems to have solved the problem of combining a foolproof one-way valve with sublime simplicity. They're made of titanium alloy and woven dacron—a sort of ball-valve, with the ball about the size of a Malteeser. And they cost a hundred and thirty quid each, which means I'll be two hundred and sixty pounds better off when I come out of hospital!'

'It all seems a bit like a miracle.'

'That's what one of the house-men said. If one gets through the operation OK, and survives the dicey period which follows—then, he said, it's like watching a miracle.'

'Pat and I have booked a front seat in the stalls. Anything else you've found out?'

'They'll only be giving me mild sedation after the operation—in spite of the collision with the bus—because they have to have my co-operation to get things moving again. Which means my lungs chiefly, and that's where we could hit trouble in my bone-ridden case.'

'Your ribs?'

'Yes. But we'll cope with that one when we reach it. I'll also be on enough antibiotics for about ten days to stock a pharmacist, and within days of the op they will put me on anticoagulants, which I'll probably have to take for the rest of my life.'

'Did we once say this business was complicated? We must have been kidding. Jim, have you seen the Chaplain?'

'Yes, he's right on the ball. He's asked if I would like to be anointed on the morning of the op.'

'And you will, of course.' She shook her head wryly. 'Well, it looks as if all those things have been done which ought to have been done! How do you feel—spiritually, I mean?'

'How do I look?'

'Peaceful. And—darling, that's what I am as well: peaceful.'

The peace lasted as the week went by. On the Wednesday it was deepened. It was my brother-in-law who triggered off that particular spiritual dynamite. I was having coffee with him downstairs when he suddenly said: 'There's a chap in C2 called Roy. I wonder if you would go and see him before you're confined to your ward?'

'Who is he?'

'He lives quite near here; he's thirty-two and is married with two children. And he's got diabetes very badly.'

He lapsed into silence, staring across the big hall filled with patients, visitors and the hum of talking. Old, young, sick, well, all submerged in the curious world of hospital visiting.

'And what else?' I knew when my brother-in-law was about to make a point. He leant forward.

'Yes, what else. Last year they took his right leg off—gangrene. Three weeks ago they amputated his left.' There was a long pause. 'And last March he went totally blind when the retinas of both eyes collapsed.'

'Oh, my God', I said.

'Yes—Oh, my God. But do go and see him, he knows about you. You'll find him—remarkable could be a word to use, but it's pretty inadequate.'

'He's coping?'

'Oh yes, he's more than coping. He's running around in a wheelchair coping with other patients. Roy can cope.'

Roy was sitting in his wheelchair by a window talking to a fellow-patient when I went to C2 later that evening, gazing with sightless eyes towards the lighted mass of Maternity Block. Useless stumps rested on the chair's edge; a thin, almost transparent hand groped in my direction as I said his name. How—*how* in the name of wonder can a blind man learn to use artificial legs?

We talked for an hour, and it did not take me that long to discover what made Roy tick. He was a Christian; a man with a faith in the power of God to help and to heal which was simple and uncomplicated. He did not believe in sitting bemoaning the past, instead he looked to the always-present future and dealt with it without bitterness. When I went to bed that night I carried some words of his which have remained with me to this day. I bring them out and look at them at times when my arthritic body seems less than co-operative.

'You've got to believe in yourself *first,* then you can believe in God. If you can't have faith in the person you know best—yourself—how can you have faith in the God who made everything, including you? You've got to believe you can do something, and then God can pick you up and help you to do it!'

Two other men were being prepared for heart surgery in my room. Tom, a big, easy-tempered man from a colliery in north Warwickshire; and Ivan, a volatile Ukrainian, a refugee during his life from both Nazi German and Communist Russian persecution, but a man who had retained both his humour and his faith in humanity. Tom was to have a single valve replacement; Ivan, an enlargement made to his own damaged mitral valve. Tom was strong and tough in spirit, and determined to conquer this blankety heart nonsense which had hit him so suddenly less than a year previously. Ivan was sick; a worn-out little man with a grim history of chronic heart and lung trouble. He put himself into the hands of the doctors with the confidence of a child, but I doubt if he knew how ill he was. Communication between doctors and patient was frequently a difficult problem:

inability to articulate, the barrier of medical mystique raised by a patient between himself and his doctor, fear of asking the right questions at the right time—all these things present a formidable task to doctors needing a patient's co-operation. Never in my life have I seen doctors and nurses at such pains to make medical facts intelligible to their patients as I did in the cardiac unit of the Walsgrave Hospital. That some patients went forward to their operations with only the sketchiest idea of what was going to be done to them was assuredly not the fault of the medical team. But some patients did, and Ivan was one of them, although in his case his poor grasp of English was probably the biggest hindrance. The problem of clear communication between doctor and patient is one of the most important aspects of all medical service; but how it can be achieved with all patients all the time is something which, at present, is beyond me. If a patient wants to know the facts, and is intelligent enough to accept them, fair enough; if they do not want to know, or are unable to understand, then communication and a good doctor–patient relationship is in jeopardy from the start.

Together, the three of us went through the run-down on tests as the week passed by. We were examined by the cardiac surgeon's registrar, a young Spaniard who, it was freely said, would end up one day on the very top rung of the specialised surgery in which he was engaged. He was already immensely skilled, but he also possessed a rich fund of humour and an eye for a pretty nurse which, I quickly learnt, kept him high up on the hospital's popularity poll. His seemingly casual, easy manner with patients went down well, once again oiling the wheels of the last few days along the path to open-heart surgery. He lounged into the treatment room one day when Miss Kay, my physiotherapist, was introducing me to a respirator which she called 'Bird'. (After the name of the American manufacturer.) Each day I lay on the treatment table and breathed oxygen through Bird, so much so that following one lengthy session I felt decidedly drunk for half an hour afterwards. Miss Kay varied the breathing practice by setting Bird to breathe for me—in other words it ventilated my lungs, regularly pumping a mixture of oxygen and air into my chest, and then drawing it out again. I found it simple and pleasant, and had no qualms about having a ventilator do my breathing for me after the operation.

'The great thing you must remember,' insisted Miss Kay, 'is not to fight the ventilator. You must relax and let it do all the work—it's your lifeline after the operation, and although it's difficult to put up with it for a long period, you have got to lie quietly and let it work for you. If you get out of phase with it and try to breathe by yourself you'll run slap into difficulties. I know the post-operative ventilator is different from Bird here, but . . . .'

'What's all this about birds?' enquired a bland voice, and the registrar's face poked round the door of the treatment room.

'I'm giving Mr Ross 'Bird' instruction,' said Miss Kay, 'He . . .'

'He shouldn't need any. All self-respecting males know all about birds, probably causes a lot of heart trouble. Are you clued up on birds, Mr Ross?'

'Very.'

'There you are: a bird-watcher. Now I,' he went on, cocking an appreciative eye at Miss Kay's excellent figure, 'am a connoisseur of birds, and I do not think that miserable thing puffing oxygen all over the place is any use as a substitute for . . .'

'Doctor, will you kindly leave me to continue teaching Mr Ross how to use this bird!' said Miss Kay firmly, 'You can discuss the merits of other sorts after the operation.' She urged the grinning face of the Spaniard out of the room, and turned back to the oxygen valves. 'He's as brilliant as he's balmy,' she said cheerfully, 'which is why the surgeon wanted him for your op.'

Then there was a doctor I was to come to rely on heavily during the following weeks, the third member of the surgical team who would perform the actual operation on me. He was an Arab (we were a compact United Nations at the Walsgrave Hospital, and in far greater harmony than the other one which has its HQ in New York), and everything he did was precise, efficient and compassionate. He siphoned quantities of blood from me, kept an eagle eye on the continuing yards of electro-cardiogram trace, and generally supervised the countdown until I was safely on the launching pad. Together with the registrar and the surgeon, he would be one of the cardiac team of fifteen people who would be present in the theatre at the time of the operation. Fifteen people, of both sexes, all of whom would have a skilled, demanding job to do. All under the command of one man, a man who could not make, or allow to be made, the slightest error in judgement or performance—the man who ultimately bore the responsibility for the whole of the operation and its aftermath: the cardiac surgeon.

The more I saw of the latter the more I was sure my insistence on coming to this hospital, to be operated on by this man, was right. Rarely in my life had I felt such confidence in anyone as I did in this big, easy-mannered surgeon, who lacked any trace of the 'prima-donna temperament' so often found until fairly recently in many top-ranking consultants—indeed, temperamental stars in medicine are still far from unknown. This surgeon never spoke down to his patients, never retired behind that maddening smokescreen of medical mystique so often put up by some doctors who enjoy sitting on the pedestal erected for them by uneasy and over-awed patients. He was straightforward in all his dealing with people, universally respected by the staff, and again—something I met with in doctors and nurses over and over again—he was a man of compassion.

Later I was to learn just what a commitment this medical compassion involved. For the Arab doctor, the junior of the surgical trio, it meant sleeping on the ward after a major operation—although 'sleeping' is a misnomer if ever there was one. It meant working hours no self-respecting trade-unionist would touch with a barge-pole: twenty-four hour shifts, and seventy, eighty, ninety, even one hundred hour working weeks were not unknown. And the cardiac surgeon: at any time of the day or night he would appear on the ward when he was concerned about a particular patient. And if he had to be elsewhere he would phone up to a dozen times a day to quiz the nursing members of the team on the condition of a patient.

As for the nursing staff: what can one say about women and girls who work long hours at an exacting, exhausting job demanding super skills and care—and working for a pittance? Maybe the feeling of us who were patients was summed up in a conversation I had a few weeks after my own operation with another patient who had been operated on for the removal of one of his lungs. David had been a working man all his life; he was a clear and logical thinker, an active member of his own trade union, and had seen his share of strikes and working to rule. Nevertheless, when one more in the long line of interminable industrial strikes hit the city of Coventry while we were both in hospital, he was nothing if not forthright in his views . . .

'I'd like to get all these b . . . s who are demanding an extra ten quid a week,' he stated vehemently, 'And have them in this unit for a few weeks—post-operative from a major lung or heart operation! And then I'd like to see all these kids who are nursing us for bloody ha'pence—the whole crowd of them—*not* turn up one morning to change dressings and give out bedpans and wash sweaty bodies. "We're on strike," they'd say, "Look after your b . . . selves!" ' He shook his head at me angrily. 'But of course they'd never do it and the public knows it. And that's why the authorities can get away with paying them wages a factory worker would laugh at—or strike over because of the insult offered them. And it's not just the nurses—look at Dr S. (the Arab doctor). Have you seen the hours he puts in? Practically on his blankety knees this morning because he's not shut his eyes properly in three nights, and the poor devil doesn't get a quarter of what most of the blokes in the factories are taking home. I'm not saying factory workers shouldn't get decent money—far from it—there's been enough exploitation in the past. But it doesn't excuse exploitation of the people who run our hospitals now! And every time industry demands another boost up in their wages, the nurses and junior doctors here get pushed a little bit further down the wages league. There's something mad in a society which lets a man who bashes pieces of metal for a living take home forty-five quid a week, while a nurse who helps keep you alive after heart surgery is lucky if she gets between fifteen to twenty quid.'

I think I would be hard pushed to find a patient who has been in a thoracic unit, or seriously ill in any hospital for that matter, to disagree with him. Money may not be the major inducement to vocational work, but nurses have to buy the essentials of life like the rest of us, and why they should be penalised because of their vocation is one of life's deeper, and more unhappy mysteries.

By the Friday evening everything was done and a peaceful, placid weekend lay before us. Confined to the ward, I spent much of the time reading, but the routine was broken on the Sunday afternoon when Jo brought the children in to see me.

It was a happy, achingly vivid interlude, and I shall not quickly forget my feelings as I saw them disappear into the lift at the end of their visit. My heart was bumping painfully as I wandered back down the ward, but I did not mind. A large part of my resolve to have this operation was because of Jo and the children—whatever my thoughts and feelings about my own future living or dying, the overwhelming determination to fight for them with every mental and spiritual resource I possessed was paramount. A bitter-sweet visit and a straining heart only underlined this resolve.

At 8.30 on the Monday morning Tom was taken to theatre for his operation. Two hours later a male nurse descended on me with clippers and razors and I was rendered as hairless as a new-born babe. In deference to my protests a miserable scrap of beard was left on me, to be removed before I went to bed that night. It was a pale shadow of its former glory, but at least Jo and Pat would be able to recognise me when they visited during the evening.

An hour later I was enjoying a glass of Guinness when a sister I did not recognise came into the room and over to my bed. She was young, small, attractive and bore an air of quiet, but definite authority. She also looked tired. She sat down and looked at me quizzically.

'I'm the ward sister on A3', she said. 'When you come round after your operation you'll find me looking after things. I thought I'd like to introduce myself, and find out if you have any questions you would like to ask me. Anything at all you feel uncertain about?'

'I've been very well briefed' I answered, liking this quiet woman immediately. 'But thanks for asking—you're in charge of super-intensive?'

'I'm in charge of the ward, but I'll be in super-intensive from the moment you come back from theatre. It's a pretty busy time for both of us.'

'That I have gathered! Yes, there is one question I've been meaning to ask—I've been asking questions all the week, so why stop now?—how many pints of blood do you transfuse over this op? I've heard rumours it's a good many.'

'We lay in twenty pints for you, to be well on the safe side, but shouldn't use anything like that. Maybe a dozen, although a lot of that will be used actually during the operation. Anything else?'

'Yes, I'll be fairly well pole-axed for the first few days following the op, right?'

'Well, yes.'

I grinned at her and stroked my mutilated beard. 'Then let it be known that anyone who touches my face with a razor while I'm unable to defend myself will also be pole-axed later on! OK?'

She laughed. 'OK. We had already heard you held strong views regarding your beard.' She held out her hand: 'Good luck, I'll see you tomorrow after the operation.'

Tomorrow. The time was racing by but the peace only grew more secure. Around tea-time I heard that Tom had come through his operation, and was now in super-intensive. Thank God for that. He had gone into his fight at fifteen stone, a big handicap for both him and the surgeon. I was heading towards mine at a sylph-like weight of eight and a half stone which, in theory at least, should be an advantage.

Eight o'clock, and Jo and Pat arrived to see me. Jo was remarkable: strong and calm, with her emotions well under control. She brought me one perfect red rose, and a slim-stemmed vase to hold it. She placed it on my locker, a symbol of the will to live and the peace which now held us both so strongly. And Pat—Pat was the calm, serene anchor we had come to value so much in months now past. Each one of us had committed the next day to God, and we were content to leave it all in his hands.

At ten o'clock (smoothly shaven for the first time in twenty-two years!) I went to bed and to sleep. I said no prayers, they would have been an intrusion on the silence. Only as I slipped off to sleep did I find my mind slowly saying the twenty-third psalm: that rock which has supported so many people in the tale of the centuries since it was written.

'Nil by mouth after midnight', read the notice on the end of my bed, so trying to ignore the early morning cups of tea, I had a leisurely bath at 7 a.m., dutifully covered my hairless body with a special cleansing cream, and went back to bed. It was made up for surgery, cot sides up, and the covers folded into a neat, if uncomfortable pad. The night staff-nurse appeared, briskly shoved two pre-med needles into my bottom, and advised me to relax and try to sleep. As she left, John, the Chaplain, arrived.

Anointing is a very ancient practice in the Church of God. There is nothing magical or supernatural about it, and it is not (or should not be) particularly associated with 'last rites', as so many people imagine it to be. I look upon it as a sacrament indicating the binding together of God and man. Now, in this fragment of space and time, God was binding together with himself a surgeon, a highly trained medical team, and myself. I lay quietly when John left the ward, and let the peace take complete possession of me.

8.30, and sister and a theatre assistant wheeled my bed out of the room, down the ward, past other patients emerging from the day-room and their breakfast, past their out-stretched hands and good wishes. Across the hub, under an illuminated sign which firmly stated No Admittance, and into the theatre unit. The chief anaesthetist and his assistants, all masked and gowned in grey, greeted me quietly, and at once got down to business. I was lifted off the bed onto a trolley (or table, I've no real idea which), and the two assistants started working on my outstretched arms. The anaesthetist loomed over me, a heavy mask in his hand.

'OK, Mr Ross, I'm going to give you some oxygen to start with. Just breathe deeply.'

The smell of rubber on my face as the mask is pressed home. The knowledge that an irreversible decision has become reality. The sight of Jo's face, and those of the children vividly before my eyes.

'Right. Now I'm going to feed in the anaesthetic.'

The old familiar pounding in my chest as the heart comes under strain. The blinding awareness that the Now is slipping away and that a mysterious, unknowable journey is beginning. The diminishing echo of clear-cut words in my mind:

'Jesus, come with me . . .'

7

RAZOR'S EDGE

Out of the nothingness a circle of light appeared. Brilliant, shining down onto my face from an unknown distance above me. No feelings, no movement, no being; only the light and the sensation of wakefulness.

An immensely tall figure moved into the circle; capped and gowned in grey; heavily masked. Into the non-being dropped a voice I had once heard an aeon of time ago . . .

'. . . round, he's coming rou . . . coming round . . . he's . . . round . . . coming . . . he's coming rou . . . '

And the figure and the light vanished. The nothingness regained possession, and I ceased to exist.

No sight, no feeling, no movement. Only a voice. Blackness only a degree less than the nothingness pressed all around me. I had no body, no knowledge. Only a voice coming from nowhere, penetrating the fog which had once been my brain.

'Four pints of fresh blood . . . three of old in the fridge . . . close eye on that bleeding, bleeding, bleeding . . . '

And the blackness remained, but one minute corner of it was lifted. I knew the voice. Had heard it before—before what? Before when? Four pints of fresh blood: for me. But why? And bleeding. I was bleeding? Why? Why should I be bleeding? Why . . .

An unbelievable pain ripped across my body, and I was awake. Someone was jerking something connected to my diaphragm. An intolerable, rhythmical movement which wrenched me out of the blackness into momentary vivid awareness of my surroundings. With eyes totally lacking understanding I looked down my body. Naked, bloody, tube-infested. Two thick tubes sprouting from my middle; someone leaning over them, pulling on them as a farmer pulls on the udders of a cow. Tubes snaking down into both arms, one clear and shining, one as red as the blood on my chest. Another tube emerging from my penis, long and obscene, disappearing into the darkness on the periphery of vision. A tube somehow protruding from the side of my throat. More tubes—no, strings?—cables?—leads, of course, leads trailing from that blood-drenched chest to some machine remote from body and knowledge.

But there was another tube. God! A monstrous tube rammed into my open mouth, down my throat and into the depths of my body. I twisted my head against it, gagged, and tried to speak. Nothing. No sound at all. No voice—no means of communicating! Panic beat a rapid tattoo inside my head and I tried to lift myself up. And a familiar face swam into my field of vision; a dark, Arab face I knew and trusted. His voice came to me clearly, shattering the nightmare of non-knowing.

'You're all right, Mr Ross. Everything is going well. You've come through the operation splendidly.'

Of course, the operation. So I was through it. They'd cut my heart open and put in some new valves. Who had? I couldn't remember, but it didn't matter. Now I'd got the bad period to cope with, but that could wait. I was too tired. Immensely, uncontrollably tired. Tubes, blood and figure tilted and slipped back into the darkness.

Two faces I knew and loved were leaning over me. Two names burst up through the clouds of amnesia: Johanna and Pat. They were smiling at me, looking at me, loving me.

'We're with you, darling, all the time.'

'We love you, Jim.'

'We're praying for you . . . '

No words or voice with which to answer. Only the eyes to try and convey that I understood. Praying for me? Dear Christ, yes, keep praying for me! If you don't I shall die. I have no strength of my own to fight this thing. No prayers, no will, no desire.

And yet . . . Again the agonising wakefulness as the tubes sprouting from my middle are milked. Milked? That is precisely what someone is doing. Milking long columns of blood from me into two tall containers beside the bed. Two figures in white are leaning over me, moving around in a ritual dance by the bed on which I am stretched out as though on a rack. A machine pants regularly by my side, and another window into my closed brain opens. That must be the ventilator, the respirator I was told would be doing my breathing for me when I came round. Grief, but it wasn't much like that kid-sized thing they'd had me practising on when I was in C3. That one—what had someone called it? A bird—that had been simple. This was a choking column thrust down my throat, and a regular pulsating which filled and emptied my lungs like a well-ordered bellows. Don't fight it! Someone had said that—sometime—somewhere. Don't fight it: let the ventilator do all the work.

Lying back, struggling to relax. All right, I won't fight it. But—I must fight something. No prayers, no will, no desire: maybe, but there was something to fight therefore there must be something left in this shell which was me which would fight. What, I didn't know, but it didn't matter. A long, long way away the familiar voice was saying something about resting for the night. There was gentle movement at the tube going into my neck. The darkness returned.

It was light when I awoke. Patches of thick fog still swirled in my brain, but I was aware. Aware of my surroundings; aware I was in the super-intensive care ward; aware of tubes and machines, nurses and doctors—and pain. Aware, above all, of the ventilator still pushed down my throat, and my inability to utter a single sound.

Intense, drenching heat soaked my body in sweat, and from somewhere a rapid clicking wormed its way into my passive mind. Regular, even, like a noisy alarm-clock bent on getting through a week in the course of a day. With the beginning of understanding my eyes shifted to the monitor standing on my left. Across its glowing face a jagged line of light zig-zagged its way. Rapid, regular, even, and as I watched the clicking sound synchronised with my sight. It was my heart I was hearing. Someone had told me that my new valves would click, and my God they were clicking! Not only clicking but drumming in my chest at a speed which seemed to shake my entire body. I tried to move; tried to call out to one of the figures moving beyond the bed to come and slow the thing down, but no sound came and I was nearly sick as the ventilator was pulled in my throat. A torrent of panic swept down through my mind. I was trapped! Couldn't move; couldn't cry out; couldn't breathe; couldn't do anything to fight off these terrible machines of which I was now part. I jerked my head frantically, and a sister I dimly recognised was leaning over me, searching me with her eyes.

'What is it, my dear?' she asked quietly.

Again I jerked my head, then with enormous labour brought my hand up to my mouth and touched the tube sticking out of it.

'Is it uncomfortable?' She moved it gently in my throat and I struggled against the intolerable inability to speak, my breathing erratic and dis-jointed.

'Don't fight the ventilator—let it breathe for you. We'll take it out as soon as possible.'

Don't fight the ventilator. Again, someone had said that to me in the remote past. What did they mean? How not fight this monster choking all my efforts to speak and breathe? Again I brought my hand up to my mouth, jerking in slow motion at the offending tube.

Sister called behind her and another nurse appeared. A pad of writing paper was put in front of me and my fingers wrapped round a pencil.

'Try and write down what you want', said the voice beside me.

Slowly, unevenly, like an old enfeebled man, I managed to scrawl a brief message:

'Tube making me feel sick.'

'We'll take it out later, but it must stay where it is for the moment. The ventilator is doing your breathing for you. It's helping you, so try and relax and don't fight it.'

Again I grasped the pencil as another intolerable thought hit my confused brain. God, I was thirsty! How long since I had last had something to drink? I must have some water—now. But how to write it down when already the pencil was slipping out of my fingers? Somewhere beyond the fog some memory stirred and I reached out for the pad. Sister held it steadily in front of me.

'H_2O.' For a moment sister stared at the scrawl, then shook her head.

'When the ventilator comes out, my dear. I know you must feel terribly thirsty but you're being given plenty of liquid through the drip. Directly the ventilator is removed I'll give you a proper drink. Now, I must deal with your drainage tubes again. Just lie quite still and try to relax.'

I lay quietly, trying to ignore the tube in my throat, the insistent demand of my senses for water, the pulling at my quivering diaphragm. The panic had subsided, but in its place I became aware of a weakness which was so overwhelming it seemed to render me less than human. Impossible to do anything in the face of such weakness. Impossible to breathe, to resist pain, to be. Impossible . . .

But somewhere there was a blind man with no legs. Somewhere beyond the fog and the unknowing was a pale, sick face looking at me with sightless eyes. Words spoken in a quiet, firm voice by a man with a destroyed body and no future drifted down to me across the chasm which divided 'then' and 'now'.

'You've got to believe in yourself *first*, then you can believe in God.'

Who had said that? Oh yes, a blind man with no legs. How, *how* did a blind man learn to walk on artificial legs? God only knew, but that blind man was determined to. 'You've got to believe in yourself . . .'

The pulling on the tubes stopped, and with the words of a blind man in my brain I slipped back into the darkness.

Time had no meaning. Reality became two efficient, compassionate sisters, one or other of whom was constantly by my side; the familiar face of the Arab doctor whose name I could not remember; and the appearances of Johanna and Pat. Where they came from, how they appeared when life seemed most insupportable, I did not know. And it did not matter. Vaguely I began to understand that a fight had been joined in which we were all engaged—doctors, nurses, Jo, Pat and myself. By their brief visits to my bedside the latter two somehow gave me strength to—if not fight, because I was too weak and confused consciously to do that for long—at least to respond to the non-stop administrations of the nursing staff. Into my muddled brain the realisation gradually seeped that these nursing sisters, with infinite skill, were hauling me along a razor's edge on one side of which stood life, and on the other death.

Drifting in and out of consciousness, my mind and memory clouded with amnesia, my body one raw, pulsating nerve-end—nevertheless I sensed that this fight was one which I alone could not possibly win. Only by the combined efforts of this extraordinarily devoted team and those who were praying for me could I emerge from the valley in which I was now wandering.

Valley? Surely I had heard something before about a valley? The ventilator shifted slightly in my throat, and again I choked. The tubes into my diaphragm were milked regularly, rhythmically. The monitor flickered rapidly by my side. The faces of Jo and Pat came and went. Valley?

A long time ago before—before when?—I had known something which had helped. Which had meaning now as I lay helplessly in my web of tubes and machines. I struggled against the mists, and again a small shutter lifted in my mind. I heard or saw familiar words appearing from an unguessable distance . . .

'. . . He restoreth my soul,

'He leadeth me in paths of righteousness, for his name's sake.

'Yea, though I walk through the valley of the shadow of death, I shall fear no evil, for thou art with me . . .'

Always with me. Even as I walk now with death as my other companion, you are always with me. And because you are, I refuse to turn onto the easier path down which death is beckoning. Vaguely my eyes return to the blood-soaked dressing stretching down my chest. Such a little calvary! No, I shall fear no evil, but stay very close. I am stripped of everything I have ever used as a defence against the troubles and the agonies of this world. I am one small prostrate human who has no existence or meaning outside of

God. Of myself, by myself, through myself I am nothing and can do nothing. I am stretched out on the borderline between life and death, and only by clinging fast to you can I know life. And life in this humanity I must retain for reasons my dulled brain cannot as yet grasp. But I must choose life! I must accept the weakness, the pain, the helplessness. I must accept the ventilator panting steadily into my chest. And I must accept the blackness . . .

But the blackness was growing less. More and more I was becoming conscious of the here and now—the immediate now, because my memory of people and events before the operation, outside the tight, enclosed world of the super-intensive ward, was almost non-existent. Almost, but not quite. I knew that a moment had to come when I would be taken off this relentless ventilator, when my lungs would have to take over and do their own work. From the past some vague memory—a voice?—surely a woman's voice?—told me that this would be a moment of crisis. Of course, during the operation I had been on the heart-lung machine, the by-pass as they called it, which meant that my lungs had been out of action for some hours. They were now filled with muck and blood and I would have to make them work on their own when they took this loathsome tube out of my throat. Well, take the thing out, and let's have a go!

Three more times I managed to scrawl on sister's pad the message 'Take this thing out!' and each time she assured me that the ventilator would be removed directly the surgeon gave the word. And suddenly the Arab doctor was by my side and the tube on which I was rapidly developing a fixation was gone. I gulped at the air with mouth wide open, suddenly aware that my chest felt as if it had been hit by a ten-ton lorry, and sister slipped an oxygen mask onto my face. I relaxed. Breathing was a labour which reduced me to new depths of weakness, but at least *I* was making my lungs move in and out and not some unmentionable machine.

'And I think the drainage tubes, sister, the transfusion tube, and the central venous pressure line in his jugular—they can all come out now.' He beamed down at me, satisfaction all over his face: 'You're doing very well, Mr Ross, keep it up!'

I opened my mouth and made an experimental noise like a pig with a sore throat. The whole of the inside of my neck was so bruised and swollen it was almost as impossible to talk as when the ventilator was in.

'May I have some water?' I got out at last.

'A little.'

A small medicine glass of water was brought and sister held it to my lips. With great difficulty I swallowed half of it, then lay back exhausted but triumphant. Once again consciousness came and went; Johanna and Pat appeared and disappeared; and movement continued on and around my body.

Sister and a staff-nurse were leaning over me. 'We're going to take these drainage tubes out—you'll be far more comfortable.'

I watched them prepare two thick pads of dressing, press them down over the tubes where they disappeared into my diaphragm—there was a quick rip, and I was gaping in astonishment at several inches of bloodied tubes in the sister's hands.

'Where on earth did all that lot go to?' I asked.

'Into your heart. But the bleeding has eased now so out they come. And tomorrow we shall move you out of here into intensive care.'

'OK. Sister, how long since I had the op?'

'Yesterday.'

'Only yesterday! Seems like a month. What's the matter with my memory?'

'You've got partial amnesia—the result of being on the by-pass machine. It'll come back.'

'Does it last long? I can hardly remember a thing.'

'A week if you're lucky.' She grinned at me: 'Sometimes up to six months.'

'To hell with that for a lark! I can't even remember what we were talking about a minute ago.'

'Your memory.'

'Oh Lord!' I looked at her closely. Almost every time I had woken up since the operation she had been somewhere within a tight radius of the bed. Surely she was the sister who had come to see me before the operation when I was still in C3? The sister who had wanted to know if I had any questions, if I had been thoroughly briefed on what to expect after the operation. She looked tired, but for some reason I expected her to. 'Do you ever go off duty?' I asked.

'Oh yes, but when I'm on duty my place is in super-intensive—with you.'

The blackness was creeping back again, exhaustion dropping in a thick blanket over my body and mind. The figure beside me wavered, and I tried to remember what we had been talking about. Then it was gone, lost in the haze of tiredness and pain which again took control of everything. But even in the confusion one tiny corner of my mind remained aware.

Aware of a skilled, compassionate team working on my body. Remotely aware of an ocean of prayer upon which I drifted like a piece of flotsam. Aware of a valley stretching out before me, dim, shadowy and fearful.

But aware, even on the razor's edge, that I was not alone.

8

OUT OF THE VALLEY

Two days after the operation I was moved out of super-intensive. Physically my body was holding its own, though a heart-rate of around one hundred and forty, together with a temperature wandering in the 105° Fahrenheit region, did not exactly encourage false optimism. And I was muddled, badly confused in my mind, subject to hallucinations and periods of agitation.

The night before I was moved, the second since the operation, I had been unable to sleep, dominated by the rapid clatter of the hard-working heart within my chest. Gradually I became obsessed with the delusion that the entire staff were conspiring against me. They loomed around, dark sinister figures intent on tormenting my body. Then a new thought hit me: they were going to tie me down on the bed; they had a rope just outside my field of vision and they were going to lash my chest fast to the bed and so keep my heart quiet. They were mocking me, concentrating on my discomfort, subtly torturing me with innuendo and suggestion, before physically attacking me. For an unknown length of time I lay fearful and straining to fight off the attack when it came. Then I could bear it no longer, and half lifting myself on the bed I shouted across the ward:

'Do it! Just try it, and I'll see you're all reported to Matron in the morning!'

A surprised night sister appeared at my side.

'Now, what's the matter? Lie back, you're getting yourself all hot and bothered. But—try what?'

'I know you're going to do it! You've got it hidden! Don't think because I'm ill I don't know! Don't . . . '

I was still shouting. She pressed me gently back onto the bed. 'My dear, no one's going to do anything. Just lie quietly and try to go to sleep.'

Sleep, that was a joke! But confusion swept over me and sister faded from view. Probably I did sleep. Much later I was interested to learn that the night report contained this comment:

'Patient had rapid heart rate and high temperature throughout the night. At one period he became highly agitated and shouted a variety of odd comments at the staff. By morning he was quite rational again, and insisted on apologising to the sister for being rude.'

Not without cause from what I remember.

The agitation returned as the morning passed. Another patient was brought into super-intensive, and my cloudy brain slowly realised that a whole team of doctors and nurses were working on her. And again hallucination took possession of my mind.

'They' were doing terrible things to this poor helpless patient who, some echo from the past told me, had just had a similar operation to my own. 'They' were tormenting her with tubes and machines and some frightful treatment designed to make her lungs work on their own. Worse still, they intended doing the same atrocities to me.

In an agony of apprehension I watched Johanna and Pat come to my bedside.

'They're going to do it to me so you can't stay long.' I stumbled over the words in my urgency to get them out.

'Do what, darling?' Jo's face was anxious as she leant over me.

'I don't know, but they're going to do it later. They won't let you stay. It's very involved and drastic.'

Jo and Pat exchanged glances. 'Look, my dear, I'll talk to sister, but try and forget it for the moment. How do you feel?'

'Hot. And this bloody heart is going like a dingbat. But they're going to do something to me and they won't let you stay.'

Up and down like a curtain went my awareness. I swam through the fog of amnesia, occasionally breaking through into light to record the 'now' with distorted clarity. But the agitation remained.

Then a group of sisters and nurses were lifting me with infinite care off the post-operative cardiac-bed, and placing me on a far more comfortable ward bed. And I was being wheeled out of super-intensive into the four-bed intensive-care room next door. A monitor was set up beside me, an electric fan placed on a locker to play its cooling stream onto my heated body, a trolley laden with instruments was wheeled up and the curtains pulled around my bed.

The Arab doctor leant over me. 'Over on your side, please Mr Ross, I'm going to relieve some of that pressure in your lungs.'

My confusion grew. With it the agitation. 'How are you going to relieve the pressure?' I mumbled. 'I've got piles, you know, you'll have to be careful.'

There was a moment's silence, then behind me I heard a nurse giggle. The doctor's voice was bland when he answered.

'My friend, I'm not prodding anything into that area of your anatomy, my interest lies only in your back. I'm going to aspirate you—remove some of the fluid from your lungs. Now, a prick while I give you a local anaesthetic and that's all you will feel.'

And it was. As he slowly drew off a considerable quantity of frothy red liquid from my lungs, I felt relief spreading all through me. The pressure and pain in my chest slackened. Breathing became easier, and the agitation in my mind died.

'Better,' I whispered as he finished, 'much better.'

'Lie still and try to sleep.' He left me, the curtains were pulled back, and I looked round the small room for the first time.

It was a room like the one I had been in on C3. And in the bed alongside was someone I recognised. His face burst through the fog and confusion: of course, Tom! Tom who had had his operation the day before mine. Grey, drawn and still, breathing oxygen noisily, he yet twitched his eyes round to me and his Geordie accent reached me faintly.

'I ask you! Proper cow it is, man. You all right?'

'All right. You?'

'Winning. Waterworks seized up, though. Can't remember anything. Man, I feel bushed!'

Bushed. Up and down went the amnesia, back and forth went awareness. Sweat ran off my naked body, the monitor blip moved on its swift course, the rapid click of my new valves sounded across the ward. And now a new element came into my tiny world to add a fresh burden.

Someone was standing beside the bed, smiling down at me.

'Hallo, Mr Ross, you're looking splendid. Feel like doing some coughing for me?'

Another layer of mist lifted from my brain, this time letting through a whole flood of memories. Here was a firm link with the immediate past; not only a voice I had already been hearing in my mind, but a name as well.

'Miss Kay! I feel as though the whole bally hospital has fallen on me. No!'

She sorted it out accurately. 'Your memory is improving, not the whole hospital—only the surgeon, and you'll feel a lot better when you have coughed. Now, let's get with it.'

We got with it. Over the next few days I came to dread and

yet value the visits of my physiotherapist more than I would have believed possible. Strong hands bearing down on my battered ribs, she made me do the exercises she had taught me during that ages-gone pre-operative period. And she made me cough, bringing up the muck clogging my lungs, forcing organs which had been quiescent during and since the operation get into action again.

'Cough!' Skilfully she slid a tube up my nose and down into my lungs. Menthol puffed and swirled in those outraged regions.

'Cough!'

A lady-like burp caused such agony I almost passed out.

'No, cough! You're not made of china—cough!'

I coughed. Hawking and spitting like a consumptive bent on shredding the last battered fragments of his lungs. Heart-rate zooming to outrageous speeds, sweat stripping the weight off my body almost visibly, every last square millimetre of my chest and abdomen singing a devil's chorus of pain.

'Cough!'

Leaning against Miss Kay, tears of effort and pain streaming down my face—but coughing, loudly, harshly; bloodied sputum coming from my lungs in a steady stream.

'Splendid! You're doing famously. A few more days and you'll be clear.'

Dear God, I need to be! Lying back only semi-conscious, oppressed by that damnable clicking from my heart, I sensed Johanna and Pat with me.

'I need a quiet mind', I whispered. 'Pray for a quiet mind for me. If I lose it I can't cope.'

'We'll pray, darling. Jim, hundreds of people are praying for you—all over the city and in Leamington. And literally hundreds of parishes all over the country—the letters are pouring in.'

Someone else appeared beside Jo and Pat. A big, familiar figure who had brought comfort to me more than once in the past. The Bishop of Coventry leaned over me and I felt his hands lightly on my head.

Quietness and healing. They swept over and through me like a flood. Despite my confusion I became aware again, this time with absolute conviction, that two factors were dragging me away from death towards life. On one hand was the constant, never-failing care of the medical staff: surgeons, doctors, sisters, nurses, physiotherapists; all backed up by the complex scientific organisation of a super-modern hospital. On the other hand, and inextricably tied to it, the strength which came to me from a non-stop outpouring of prayer from family, friends, and total strangers. Weak and muddled though I was, I knew that both factors were vital to my very life. Without the medical team hauling me across the post-operative battlefield I was utterly lost. And without the prayers and support of these other countless friends I was also lost, because if once my will to live collapsed I would be unable to co-operate with the medical team. And then I would die.

'Yea, though I walk through the valley of the shadow of death, I shall fear no evil, for thou art with me . . .'

Like a drowning man I clung onto the anchor I knew. And the anchor never slipped.

They were sponging down my heated body when I asked sister the question that had been with me all day.

'Sister, how's Ivan?'

She looked at me for a long time without answering as she dried my outstretched arm. Then:

'Ivan died. I'm so sorry—he didn't survive the operation.'

So Ivan had gone. Three of us had been prepared for open-heart surgery in our room on C3 during that pre-operative period. And we had all been told the risks. But Ivan had died while I had lived.

Again the Bishop was beside me. 'Ivan,' I said, 'Why did it have to be Ivan?'

His hands were smoothing my hair, quieting, calming. 'Ivan is all right. We must pray for his widow . . .'

Yes, his widow. So easily it could have been Johanna who was the widow. My children who had lost their father. What had the surgeon said to me all those weeks ago? Fifty per cent. Your chances of coming through this are possibly fifty per cent. *But without the operation there was no chance at all.*

I looked up at the Bishop. 'Can't remember much,' I said slowly, 'But there's something in the Bible somewhere which says—"Unto whom much is given, much shall be asked"—something like that, anyway. I know what it means now. There's a lot to do in the future—got to write a book about all this lot. I've got to let people know about the fantastic work the team here does—not just to me, but every week! Regularly. On dozens of people who haven't got the ghost of a chance of living without them. And I've got to write about this miracle of prayer. You know better than anybody how heavily I've slammed the institutional Church in the past: but it works! Despite all its mucking about with worn-out buildings and talking shops and archaic stupidities, there's still a rock-steady centre of it which works! In spite of all its cock-eyed committees and synods and piddling closed-shop lunacies—it still works! One of its members is in extremis and hundreds of ordinary little churches all over the place simply pray for him, and that prayer works!' I lay back, exhausted by my outburst: 'It's a damned silly Church, and it's wasting a lot of its time and most of its opportunities, but it is still the Church of God. And those people who would like to get rid of it all—buildings, priests, congregations, committees and all the rest of it—are wrong. Because underneath all the clutter it's still the Church of Christ, and it works. I know, because I wouldn't have had the will to live without it.'

The Bishop held my hands tightly. 'You'll write that in a book? It's important, because I think this is the only hope some people have got.'

'Yes, I'll write it.' When I'm stronger. When the weakness goes. When the amnesia which blurs even the familiar face of the Bishop has gone. When I step out of this valley.

As I am going to.

Five days from the operation and my memory beginning to clear. It was Sunday and John brought Holy Communion to me early in the morning.

'Can you come more than once a week?' I asked him. 'I'm not out of the wood yet and I need a lot of help. I've no strength, and not much will.'

'I'll bring you the Sacrament three times a week. Will that be OK?'

Yes, that would be OK. Ever since I had been a Christian the Holy Communion had been the focus of my faith. I was too worldly, I had been an agnostic for too great a proportion of my life, to take easily to a conventional Christian discipline. Over the years many of my friends had considered—and called me—frivolous about my faith, but the hope and joy in Christianity has always rung a greater bell with me than negative strictures and harping on sin. We are all sinners—selfish, bungling, egotistical sinners prone to hurt our neighbours and ourselves by our damn-fool antics: of course we are. Christians or not, we are all tarred with the same brush.

But if we really try to be Christians—followers of a crazy man who once wandered about a tin-pot, fiddling little Middle-eastern state spreading joy, compassion and healing —if we try to follow the ways of that man who in some mysterious manner can still accompany one today even through the trauma of open-heart surgery if we will let him—then the main characteristic one is going to catch from that man is joy.

And to keep that man who is God in my sights and to catch the infection of his joy, I, fallible and not at all at home with many of the man-made dogmas and dictums we have hung onto the Christ, I must have the focus of his Holy Communion.

'OK,' said John, 'Three times a week.'

Part of the meaning of Holy Communion came home to me forcibly as I lay in bed later that first Sunday after the operation, trying to struggle through the exhaustion which still lay on me like a plague. There was movement at the door, a wheelchair was manœuvred to my bedside, and a blind man with no legs was groping for my hand.

'Roy!'

'Tried to get in to see you before, but they blocked me.' The sightless eyes were fixed on my face, and he nodded slowly. 'You're nearly through it, aren't you?' he asked quietly.

'Nearly. It's been a bit of a journey.'

'Yeah, but you had a lot of company.' Suddenly he grinned: 'I can hear your new valves—how do they feel?'

'They're beginning to slow down, Roy . . .' I paused, groping for words to express something I knew, suddenly, was very important. Overwhelmingly important—and something I had hardly realised until now.

'Roy, I've discovered a miracle', I said finally. 'For over thirty years I've hardly ever known a time when I hadn't got a pain of some sort in my heart. It's banged and thumped and gurgled, and palpitated like a clapped-out donkey engine. It's given me every unpleasant feeling in the book—and now it's all gone! All of it. Oh Lord, I think I had pain and discomfort in most parts of my body when I came round, and I still feel like two-penn'orth of cold tripe. But not in my heart! There's been no pain, no palpitations—nothing there at all except a high heart-beat since the moment I had that op. And the beat is already slowing. I've got a new heart, Roy, and it's working properly!'

'Yeah, a miracle. A medical one, and one of faith. They weren't at all sure they'd get away with it, were they, mate? Not with your spine and grotty bones. Fifty-fifty the surgeon told you—right?' He grinned at me: 'Maybe he was forgetting the X-factor.'

'I don't think he forgot even that', I replied slowly, thinking of what I knew and had seen of the surgeon. 'In fact, I think you'll find he took it into his calculations. I intend to ask him about that. He's awfully easy to talk to and I've a strong hunch he's a man with a faith. Anyway, I want to find out. You know I had this feeling all along that he, and no other surgeon, should do this op?'

'Even though he nearly sent you down to London?'

'Particularly because of that. When he told me the facts and the odds all those weeks ago in Outpatients at Warwick, he showed a humility I didn't think big surgeons have. And he was—diffident when he said he'd make up his mind after his team had had a go at me. Yet I could see he wanted to do it. He called it a challenge.'

'It was all of that.' Roy smiled again, his face quizzical: 'Started writing again yet, Jim?'

'Blimey, give me a chance!'

'You'll have to get this part down soon or it will fade. Suffering always does.'

I squeezed his hand. 'You should know. I'll start writing as soon as I can—give me a week or two.'

'And the X-factor? How will you deal with that?'

There was a long silence, and I glanced round the ward.

Tom was heaving his bulk out of bed, determination and effort mingled on his tough Geordie face. Diagonally across from me was a patient who was not winning his fight, a young man who had undergone precisely the same operation as myself, but for whom everything had since gone wrong: physically, mentally, spiritually. Deep in his own valley the journey for him was almost over, and there would be no ending of it in this mortality. In the bed opposite lay a man of seventy-four who had just been given a pace-maker to regulate a heart which otherwise would simply stop. Cheerful and confident, he was already sitting up and taking notice, talking with relish of getting down to his club for a beer in a couple of weeks' time. In the next room a middle-aged woman was recovering rapidly from an operation to replace her defective mitral valve. And in super-intensive another woman was fighting the aftermath of double-valve replacement, while a little girl of eight lay breathing on the ventilator; the hole in her heart skilfully mended, her future assured. And we were only one week's work in one cardiac unit similar to heart units up and down the country. True, every last one of us had faced risks, some small, some great, but without open-heart surgery the future of all of us would have been limited or nil.

'I can deal with this side of it,' I replied at last, 'But mine is a very restricted view—you know what I mean. We—you and I and all these other patients—just have to do what the doctors and nurses tell us; we have to draw on whatever spiritual resources we may or may not have—and either live or die. But it's all far more difficult for our wives or husbands to cope with. They're the ones who take the real beating at a time like this, and this is where I think the X-factor comes in.'

'Right. So?'

'So I'll have to find out what's been happening these last few days—Jo's side of things, I mean. I don't know anything except odd bits and pieces which have edged through this damned amnesia. But I'm getting better, Roy.'

'Sure you are. And I'm going to get my new legs and we'll both have a story to tell. So long, Jim. And when you write it let 'em know that having a spot of faith is all part of the medical cure.' He gripped my hand for the last time. 'Tell them that when you have the total experience you don't just believe in God. You know.'

Such a little time before Roy knew far more than I did. He never did get his legs. Only a few short weeks remained before he experienced the climax of his total experience.

It doesn't take long to die when a blind man with no legs has a massive cerebral haemorrhage.

'We're moving you.'

'OK sister—where?'

'A two-bed room just along the ward. You'll be on your own and be able to rest. You're not sleeping, are you?'

'No, it's like Piccadilly in here.'

'Well, you'll find it much more peaceful down the ward. Has Miss Kay had you up again?'

'Yes. Slow time to the fire-escape. Didn't you hear my castenets?'

'If you mean your valves—I can hear them now. Grinding in very nicely, I'd say. How's the amnesia?'

'Nearly gone.'

'Pain?'

'What pain?'

'Um. Sputum?'

'Plenty! I've become a dirty old man.'

'Miss Kay is very pleased with you. It's up to you to get rid of what's left—you don't need her help any more. How's the wound?'

'Beautiful. When are the stitches coming out?'

'Tomorrow.'

'And when are you throwing me out of here?'

'Not for at least a month. You are still very post-operative, so behave.'

'Seriously, sister, what does the surgeon think of the way things are going?'

She smiled broadly, took the brakes off the bed and started it rolling towards the door.

'He's like a dog with two tails. Why don't you ask him yourself?'

'I shall. Sister, we're out of the wood, I take it?'

'Yes, as long as you are sensible and remember that you've just had a pretty massive operation. For several months you should do practically nothing; rest a lot and give your whole body a chance to recover. It will be a year before you really begin to feel strong, and maybe three years before you get the full benefit of these new valves, but—you're going to be all right!'

Too right I was. I could feel it deep inside me, both physically and in my clearing mind; the first faint sensations of well-being stirring in my whole body. Sister turned her head sharply as we trundled down the corridor.

'What did you say?' she asked.

'I said this was some hospital.'

'You've had some surgeon, believe me.'

'I'll believe you. And if we're going to eulogise—some nurses. And sisters.'

She pushed me into a small, blissfully peaceful room, bedecked with flowers, and with a magnificent view out over Coventry.

'Yes,' she smiled, 'And one or two other factors as well.'

Which leaves me with Johanna. I have had my heart cut open, and two artificial valves made of titanium alloy and woven dacron stitched inside it. But my description of that happening has been limited and one-sided. The X-factor, without which I would have died because there would have been no will to live—that belongs to Jo.

9

THE X-FACTOR

AND I can't write! I've told Jim so dozens of times, but the only result is that I'm sitting here chewing a biro while trying to get the most vivid memories I ever have had, or ever shall have, down on paper.

Fortunately, I know my husband so well that I was certain he would be itching to get cracking on his book again directly he could hold a pen without actually dropping it. So I noted down my impressions of those incredible ten days following his operation as soon as possible after they happened. For the first week I could only watch, and wait for the outcome of the battle going on in his body. Then, as it gradually became clear that he was going to recover, I sat down one evening and scribbled down my memories—almost compulsively recording the wonder of that time while it was still vivid.

Pat helped tremendously by writing a detailed letter to Chris a couple of days after the operation. It was a wonderful letter, and Chris later sent it back to me, realising that it contained much that Jim would need for his book.

And, looking back, I think that was one of the most remarkable things about the whole affair: we *knew* Jim would continue the book he had started before the operation was even finally decided upon. In spite of all the medical risks, *he* would finish the book—this book—and it seemed irrelevant for any of us to suppose otherwise.

Once, during those endless weeks of waiting before the decision to operate was taken, he said to me: 'I haven't the slightest intention of pegging out yet, either from another heart attack or on an operating table, but if the good Lord does have other ideas—then you'll have to finish the book. It can still help, because people are often so afraid! Afraid of death, afraid of dying, afraid of suffering. So terribly afraid of the unknown. And there's no need to be at all: life is only a school, and suffering, dying and death are lessons of no greater or lesser importance than joy, happiness or loving. So don't leave the book unfinished, love, because it can still have quite a lot to say whether I type The End or not. I intend to write that last chapter, but you may have to. Don't forget to use a dictionary—your spelling is even worse than mine!'

By the grace of God I am not writing the last chapter, only the next to last. And although I find writing for publication a pretty nerve-racking business, I think Jim is right in insisting I do this. What Pat and I experienced, mentally and spiritually, should be told, because I doubt if either of us will ever again know such a deep and constant communion with God. What follows now is brief, sketchy and bald, but it is hardly altered from the two accounts which Pat and I wrote down while the actual events were happening. I have dovetailed together Pat's letter to Chris and my own notes: the result may not have great literary merit, but it does recount what was to us, and to many, many others, a modern miracle.

I don't have to try very hard to take my mind back to that last day before the operation . . .

It was a quiet day, with no worries and no fears. All the tensions and looking forward of the past months were gone. I don't think I have ever felt so calm, even though I was tremendously conscious of being caught up in something which had got to a point where nothing I could do would alter or stop it. For nearly seven years I had lived with the knowledge that Jim's diseased heart could leave me a widow at any time: now we had come to the crisis and I was sure we would come through it to a new life together. Besides, it made no sense at all to me for God to let Jim die on an operating table after giving him the strength to keep alive thirty years longer than any doctor had said was possible. But it did make sense for him to survive this operation. There was so much mystery and fear about heart surgery, so much nonsense spoken by moralists and self-styled experts on the whole subject of medical transplants and replacement surgery. Jim *had* to survive the operation—he was a writer, and it was his job to debunk some of this nonsense, his task to state from the patient's point of view just what medicine and faith together can achieve in this age of scepticism—and seeking. Cold logic said that within twenty-four hours I could well be a widow, but logic can disappear like mist under sun when the calm of faith prevails.

Pat arrived from Bristol around five o' clock, and at seven-thirty we left for the hospital. We found Jim in the same mood of calm as ourselves—only grieved (aggrieved!) at the loss of twenty-two years growth of beard. 'It's not the surgeon,' he mourned, 'He can do his plumbing whether the beard is there or not. It's the ruddy anaesthetist—insists there could be difficulties with masks and tubes with fungus still on my face. But, I ask you—twenty-two years pruning and beaver-culture gone in a few minutes. It's flaming sacrilege!'

We stayed an hour. Only as we left did the wild unreality of the situation rise inside me, but . . . 'Bring in some Scotch to pour down my drip tomorrow,' he said, 'Or maybe not tomorrow, better leave it a couple of days. And look after the children.'

We did not leave the hospital immediately, but went up to the chapel on the top floor—a trip we were to make many times in the following days. In that beautiful, peaceful place

Pat and I prayed together, and I made the final decision to give Jim to God without any strings at all attached. If God gave him back to me so that we might know the joy of more years together in this mortal part of life, then—thanks be to God. And if God decided otherwise, still—thanks be to God. There is only one life, after all, and the veil of death does not divide for long.

We got up early for what was to prove the longest day of my life. The calm was still there as we dressed the children, had breakfast and got Jonathan off to school. And it remained as the morning started to pass, but again the unreality gripped me as we got on with ordinary household chores. At nine o'clock I phoned the hospital, and was told that Jim had been taken to the theatre at half past eight. The operation had got under way immediately, and now we could only wait and pray.

In her letter Pat wrote: 'It really was the most fantastic day. We seemed to be held calm in the centre of a whirlpool —conscious of calm and peace and serenity all through the long eight hours of the operation. Only when the phone rang, as it did many times, was this calm shattered and our hearts leapt into our mouths. Then we would realise how precious was this calm, and how disastrous the fear which lay beyond it. Again and again we managed to regain this calm by sitting down quietly in prayer and meditation, and each time we valued more the peace which was being given to us. Over and over again we were conscious of the prayers and love of people holding Jim up, and keeping us calm.'

Without prayer, and without the strength and support of Pat, the day would have been intolerable. I remember sitting in the kitchen with her in the afternoon, and praying for the calm to remain with us as the hours ticked away and the stream of telephone calls continued. So many calls, but nothing from the hospital. Only the silence which had lasted all day, and was unchanged when Johnny arrived home from school. The surgeon had promised to phone directly the operation was over, and I knew he would not let us down. But so much time was passing, and at four o' clock I could bear it no longer. Charlotte arrived, the friend who was to baby-sit for us, staying the entire night or as long as was needed should circumstances prove it necessary, and at last I phoned the hospital, only to learn that Jim was still in the operating theatre.

It was impossible to stay at home any longer, because after so long it was also impossible to stop the rise of tension inside us, and we all knew how easily that sort of thing could communicate itself to the children. Nearly eight hours had passed since the operation began, and we had been told it should take about six: fear was still absent, but I began to feel sick and distressed at the knowledge that this massive surgery on Jim was still going on.

Pat packed our overnight case and we left, but did not go directly to the hospital. Instead we stopped at the parish church to kneel in the pew which Jim and the children and I occupied each Sunday at family Communion. And again we found peace, and the courage to drive to the hospital and into the unknown.

We arrived at 5.15 and went straight to A3. We were told that Jim was just back from the theatre and was more or less conscious. For a few moments we had to wait outside the super-intensive care room, and there beside us was Jim's locker, his slippers on it—so intimately his, and so achingly empty. But on top of the locker was the single red rose I had given him the night before: still blooming, still perfect, and still living.

Hand in hand, Pat and I went in to see him. We stayed only a couple of minutes and said something—what, I cannot remember. Jim nodded slightly; he could not speak because some large tube was coming from his mouth, pulling it right down on one side. I can't even try to pretend he did not look terrible—he appeared to lie in the middle of a mass of tubes and machines. Almost, I felt, he was part of a machine, and I knew a sense of shock, became cold and felt very sick.

And there was blood—everywhere it seemed to our shocked eyes. We had been warned that he was bleeding; indeed, the operation would have been over a couple of hours earlier had he not started a severe haemorrhage from the wound. Later we learnt that he had actually come round for a few seconds on the operating table: to all intents and purposes the operation had been finished and the flow of anaesthetic was being stopped. Then came the haemorrhage and the whole chest had to be re-opened, examined, and painstakingly sutured again. Yet the eyes which looked back at Pat and me were the same eyes I had known for seven years, with the same warmth and love.

Shaken, Pat and I were shown to the room at the end of the ward where we were to spend the night. And again we prayed, tremendously grateful that Jim had come through the first ordeal of the day-long operation, but acutely aware that his life now rested on the finest of balances.

A little later, after spending a short time in the chapel, we slipped out for an hour to Jim's sister who lived a few miles away, where we were dosed with large glasses of sherry and made to eat a meal. By nine o'clock we were back at the hospital, waiting at the nurses' station on A3 to go in and see Jim again.

Suddenly a sister came out of super-intensive and went to the phone—she wanted a doctor urgently, the drainage tubes from Mr Ross's heart were blocked, would the doctor come immediately? I stopped her as she was walking quickly back and asked her what was the matter. Everything would be all right, she tried to reassure us, would we go to our room and we would be able to see Jim as soon as the doctor had cleared things up. As we walked down the ward we were passed by the Arab doctor hurrying towards super-intensive. Even more shaken, and with the peace gone, we went into our room.

Where I would have been without Pat I do not know. She held me as the storm of tears raged, then prayed for the peace to return. Again I must turn to her letter:

'Gradually this happened. We could feel it happening: first the tension and heart-beating diminished, and then, like water seeping up into a hole in wet sand, the peace and confidence returned. As I was giving thanks I was suddenly aware of a presence. It was like an electric shock, mainly up and down my spine but all over as well, plus a feeling of heat and greatly heightened awareness. Without knowing why, or what I really meant, I said: "Dorothy[1] is with us. Here in this room and helping us."

'The ecstasy of that awareness lasted—Oh, how long? Then I became aware that Cuthbert[2] was praying at that precise time for Jim. It was all very strange, but wonderfully helpful, and I knew that the power of God to help and heal was as strong today as it has ever been.'

A few minutes—or an age—later, a nurse appeared and said we could see Jim although he still had a considerable degree of bleeding which must be stopped. And then we were standing beside him again, holding his cold, clammy hands, telling him we loved him and were with him. For the rest of my life I shall not forget what he looked like, or the physical

[1] Dorothy Kerin, founder of the Home for Divine Healing at Burrswood in Kent. Dorothy Kerin had a great influence on the author's early Christian years, and they became very close. She died in 1963.

[2] Later we learnt that Cuthbert, the Bishop of Coventry, had been praying for Jim at that precise moment. He was then 2000 miles away in Greece.

hurt which rose inside me at the sight of so much helplessness and suffering. Yet, equally, I shall not forget the way in which he nodded when we spoke, and the expression in his eyes saying the words he could not speak.

As we left super-intensive I glanced back at him, then at Pat, and saw my query reflected in her own eyes. Had Jim a tube inserted in the front of his neck, as well as that small one going into the side of it? Had they performed a tracheotomy or not? I did not know, and for a long time back in our room could not even ask Pat, so great was the hurt within me, so tremendous the longing to take some of the burden off the man I loved, and who now lay with his body outstretched as though in crucifixion only a few yards away.

But again, out of the anguish the calm returned, and soon we were sitting together drinking tea and talking of what we thought we had just seen—or had not seen. We were both unsure of details, because we had had eyes only for Jim's face and nothing else, but we both had the impression that he had not had a tracheotomy—otherwise why was that large tube disappearing into his mouth?

At that moment Jim's brother-in-law came into the room to see us, and I asked him if he would find out definitely whether or not Jim had had a tracheotomy. Looking back it seems a small point, but at that time it loomed large. The return to normal breathing was going to present Jim with enough problems as it was: those problems would be magnified if he had to rely for his source of air on an artificial hole in the throat.

But—there was no tracheotomy. In the chapel some hours before Pat had been sure that this would be so; now we could only rejoice and feel our spirits rising that this was one less problem with which Jim would have to contend.

Incredibly, we slept that night. We knew Jim was still haemorrhaging, knew the medical and nursing teams were working non-stop on him, knew that we were caught up in a crisis which would last for days. And yet we slept. Tremendously aware of the prayers of so many people supporting us, and achingly conscious of the power of God to create wholeness out of suffering. In retrospect I sometimes wonder what the humanist, the *avante-garde* 'Christian' apologist, the cleric who explains away the Gospel's miracles in 'logical terms', and all the rag-tag-and-bobtail who ballyhoo for a rationalised Christianity 'acceptable to man-come-of-age'—I wonder just what these people have to offer suffering mankind in his moments of greatest need? Because there is only one thing which makes any sense, or offers any hope, when men and women get down to the basics of life; when they have to cope with living and loving, suffering and dying, death and the unknown beyond death.

God as a benevolent Santa Claus will not help. Neither will an emasculated Christ relegated to the banalities of sugary hymns or a watered-down Gospel. Only the fatherhood of God, as revealed by the Jesus who died a brutal death on the cross, and rose again, can help suffering mankind when the chips are really down. The God who chose to show the way of life through the path to, and the climax of crucifixion, was very close to us that night: only a God who knew intimately the trauma of suffering and dying—and resurrection—could help us. And he did.

And so, secure in the belief that our crucified Lord was pouring his own strength into the body and mind of a man who had his heart cut open, we slept.

Our belief was not misplaced.

In the chapel that Tuesday night we had prayed for two specific things: that Jim's bleeding would stop, and that the children, at home, would sleep soundly and not be too affected by the dramatic events we were all going through.

At seven fifteen on the Wednesday morning a nurse brought us tea and told us that the bleeding had stopped during the night; and a phone call home a little later reassured us about the children. As the day slowly advanced we came to know a deep joy at just how tremendous a factor —the X-factor, as Jim called it—prayer was in the whole business. The surgeon and the staff on A3 did not try to pretend to us that Jim was sailing through this critical post-operative period: every step of the way was a battle fought, and won, against heavy odds, and every step achieved was a minor advance on the road to victory. And Pat and I could only marvel at the patience, the determination and compassion which the whole medical and nursing team played in these battles.

Every step, every battle, great or small, was the subject of prayer—not just by Pat and myself, but by a close-knit team of friends and family up and down the country. And beyond them the tremendous flood of prayer from those who could not know specific details, only that the need was great and the crisis at its height. Every time a new need arose we phoned 'the team', as we called them, and the response of prayer was so immediate that every problem was overcome. The surgeon and the staff knew what we were doing, and several of them were adding their own prayers to ours: such a combination of the most advanced techniques of medical science and uncomplicated trust in God can rarely have been put to better effect.

For slowly the battle was won. On Wednesday, Jim was taken off the ventilator and most of the tubes came out: he remained incredibly weak, impossibly exhausted, yet was able to pull aside the oxygen mask and say a few words to us in a hoarse, uncertain voice. He was not very coherent and seemed to have little memory of anything, past or present, yet we could see he was struggling to throw off the amnesia and regain normal control of his senses. Everything was offered up to God in prayer: his amnesia; his very high temperature and its attendant discomfort of heat; his far too rapid heart-beat which revealed its urgency in those flickering monitor screens; his pain and discomfort, his weakness, his need for a strong will to live. His confusion on the Thursday, and the agitation he suffered before his lungs were aspirated—what he thought was going to happen to him none of us knew, but it was the one and only time we saw him distressed for himself. We did see him distressed again three days after the operation when he insisted on knowing what had happened to Ivan, and learnt he had died in the theatre; this also we offered up to God.

There are so many people who dismiss prayer and God as psychological wanderings and fantasies: let them. The loss is theirs, and they are poorly armed when they come face to face with this thing we call death. There are modern 'Christians' who reject anything supernatural in the Christian faith, who live a humanist religion and try to explain away in material terms anything that smacks of the mysterious omnipresence of God. Again—let them. The man Jesus would have no power to help and heal twentieth-century man if his roots were grounded only in first-century Galilee. The God who has been worshipped—and reviled—down through the centuries would be a pointless abstraction if the totally affected lives of untold numbers of men and women did not testify otherwise.

God is; and his power is as all-embracing now as it was for the first small group of men Jesus called his disciples. And to those who would laugh at me, I can only ask 'have you ever seen a miracle?' Because I have. The miracle of a man, badly crippled with advanced ankylosing spondylitis, a man with a hip destroyed by osteo-arthritis, a man with a rib-cage become rigid under long years of arthritic hardening, a man with two major valves in his heart totally ruined and the rest of that heart enlarged beyond all normal limits—the miracle of this man coming through major open-heart surgery against formidable odds, and then surviving the battering of his post-operative state. To all of us who watched his survival this was a miracle, and I use the word with no reserve, no apology. It was no surprise for me to learn later on that the surgeon himself was a Christian, a man of prayer, and that he had reckoned on the power of prayer—the X-factor—as one more weapon to help get his patient through the operation and the period of crisis beyond.

As long as I live I shall not forget those ten days when Pat and I watched, waited and prayed. They brought Pat and me closer than I have ever been to anyone else except Jim. And they brought me to a knowledge of the power and presence of God which I do not believe can ever fade.

I remember going to see Jim the day he was moved up the ward into a quiet room by himself. He still looked desperately tired and ill, a scrubby beard regrowing on his face (far too slowly as far as he was concerned!), the dressing still on his chest, and the clicking of his new valves greeting me as I went in the door.

But the old sparkle was back in his eyes, his memory clear and his voice firm. I knew that the future for us in this world still existed.

And the prayer in my heart became a song.

10

HEARTS ARE TRUMPS

For five more weeks I remained in hospital. Slowly gaining strength, learning to use my body again, getting used to the loud clicking from my new valves which, from now on, would be my constant companion. Slowly thinking my way through the whole experience, discovering in the process a quietness of mind of a quality I have never before known so richly.

They were weeks of tremendously mixed emotions. Of joys, happiness, and growing confidence, shared by Jo, our family and friends, the staff and myself alike; but also of the deeply sobering realisation of the fragility of the tightrope across which I had been walking, and for a long time to come, though in more minor key, I would still be walking.

Long talks with fellow-patients, nurses and doctors, confirmed in me the knowledge that no one undergoes major open-heart surgery, or is even advised to, unless the alternative prospect of living a normal life—or living at all—is bleak. That risks are involved in this type of heart surgery at the present state of medical knowledge cannot be denied, but that same surgery does offer hope of life to untold numbers of people who otherwise have little or no hope. And this is the factor which must be looked at squarely when the emotive subjects of transplant or replacement surgery hit the public awareness.

I have read so much rubbish on these subjects during the past decade! There have been so many high-flown words spoken on the morals and ethics involved in replacing someone's diseased organs by those taken from living or dead donors; or with animal or artificial organs. A whole torrent of words, and only a tiny proportion of that flood has come from those qualified to speak out on such complex subjects: doctors, surgeons, nurses, a few of the more far-seeing clergy, a smattering of people with enough vision to see beyond the surgeon's knife and the mortician's slab. But the majority of all this comment, particularly in regard to heart surgery, has come from those totally unqualified to dogmatise on such a specialised topic: a stream of ignorant and often sickeningly pious humbug from people who have not the faintest idea just how shattering to the human frame a disabled, failing heart can be.

But among all the argument, all the discussions, all the wrangling, all the expressed fears, I have not yet seen outspoken comment from the one person who is in a better position than anyone else to pass judgement on heart and replacement surgery: the man or woman who possesses a heart so damaged by disease that they walk with death as their constant companion.

Let me be quite clear about this: I am afraid neither of death nor of dying. Thirty years' coexistence with a battered heart have seen to that. I do not believe that death means the end of this thing we call life: far from it. Death is only a staging-post between one part of living and another, and the part we do not yet know I believe to be far more vital and vivid than the mortality which holds us tied to the confines of our limited, and often suffering bodies. Death is not an end: only another beginning.

And my experience of suffering and death is not confined only to my weak body; it has been my lot to witness at the closest possible range the suffering and dying of other people. At first hand I know the terrifying hurt of bereavement: the gap which becomes achingly real—almost the only reality—when someone loved is whisked away by death. I have been present at the months' drawn-out crucifixion of a child dying from a cancer so monstrous it destroyed her body before death intervened. I have held the dying in my arms, and experienced the never-to-be-forgotten trauma of feeling, sensing, the irreversible withdrawal of the personality, the spirit, the 'I' of a loved one, as the body of the beloved has become cold with the arrival of death. I have experienced the aftermath, not once but many times, and over the years I have tried to look clearly at, to understand and come to terms with this thing we who go on living call bereavement. First comes shock; urgent and panic-evoking in the case of sudden death, still painfully present although the illness and death of one's partner, child or friend has been long drawn-out. Shock which can be almost paralysing in its effect; physical as well as mental and spiritual—shock, I believe which must be similar to that suffered by a sudden, unexpected amputation. One moment the limb is there, the next it is gone. One moment the wife, husband or child is there: the next they are gone. In either case there is a sense of deprivation—mutilation even, which can be harmful to the whole human system. The only difference is that the healing of bodily amputation, with all its mental and spiritual connotations, can be far quicker than the amputation of one human being from another.

And with the shock of sudden bereavement comes the emptiness. The realisation that this moment, this hour, this day—all the tomorrows which stretch out ahead in a dreary procession must be walked without the one who has just died. That the book being read must go back to the library unfinished. The engagements cancelled. The holiday abandoned—little things, unimportant things which overnight lose their insignificance and emphasise the emptiness. I think the emptiness of bereavement is probably the most difficult consequence of all to deal with. It dominates from waking to sleeping, a chasm which sometimes seems too formidable ever to be filled.

Yet—it must be filled! If the human spirit is to be true to itself, and especially true to the one who has just died, then that shock and emptiness must be faced squarely, and conquered. With most people this happens sooner or later: an unhappy few never succeed in emerging again into the real world of living. That world, which, for those with enough faith to look for it, embraces the material world in which we now live, and the unseen world to which death is only the door. For this is at the heart of bereavement, and this ultimately is the test of a real faith: to stand firm in the desolation of human loss and say—'I know that I am not alone. I do not know how, when or where—such terms are meaningless—but I know that my Redeemer, and my love, is alive!'

This is the test of real, lasting recovery from bereavement: whether one can emerge a wiser, more adult person, or just 'get over it'. A lot of people do just that—they 'get over it'. The emptiness fills, after a fashion. The amputation heals, more or less cleanly. The pain dies, the memory dims; the face, voice and being which were once an integral part of one's whole life, blur and are lost. They get over it, take up the threads of life and, more or less, carry on with the business of living.

But more or less is not good enough. I remember vividly a good friend coming to see me soon after the death of my first wife. He had lost his own wife ten years earlier, and he was not being glib.

'In the weeks and months to come,' he said, 'people are going to say to you—"Well, old chap, time is a great healer: you'll get over it. Just give it time and you forget, you know." Or some such words, you can imagine them as well as I can. Don't take any notice of them. You're not meant to just forget it or get over it: you're meant to learn by it!'

And that, I believe, is the nub of the whole business of bereavement: we are meant to learn from it. Bereavement is inevitable. It must come to every one of us. Yet all too many people merely try to 'get over it' as quickly as possible, and resume 'normal' living. They forget that bereavement is a part of normal living.

When we, as individuals, hit the rocks of bereavement, or any suffering for that matter, we are meant to go over those rocks, and not scramble around or try to dodge them. We cannot in this life keep on avoiding the unpleasant—living, in the fullest meaning of the word, means tackling all and everything to come our way, and that includes bereavement.

It is no trite platitude, but absolute fact, to state that one cannot ever know the heights without experiencing the depths.

In exactly the same way that we are meant to learn more about life and God through joy, happiness, working and playing, so I believe we are meant to learn from those darker, but deeper things which touch every last one of us at some time or another: death, grief, bereavement. And the lesson of bereavement, if faced without prejudice or fear, leads anyone who tries to live as a Christian to one place only: the cross of Christ. And the cross leads into the very presence of God.

In the emptiness of bereavement, it is very hard to be positive, even more difficult to look out from one's own agony to that of another, and it is in this situation that friends, especially friends of faith, are beyond value. For to be taken by the hand of friendship, in faith, to the foot of the cross marks the point at which the well of emptiness begins to fill. The eternal paradox is revealed again—the bereavement still exists, the wife, husband or child is still dead. The amputation remains an amputation. But mysteriously, unanswerably, the pain of bereavement which once seemed so intolerable a burden is now shared, and has become a source of strength.

Here is the mystery and the maturity of bereavement faced in faith: if it is taken to the cross of Christ it cannot remain plain, stark, shocked emptiness. No matter how it is taken—in grief, anger, fear—as long as it is taken to the Christ of the cross, that bereavement will be transformed from negative emptiness into a positive force. Because when it is so taken, it is an admittance that I—the great, proud, ever-able-to-cope-I—can do nothing! It is a hand-over to someone who can and does do everything. Such a hand-over can be the beginning of the formation of a right relationship with God, and that, ultimately, is all that does matter in life.

To go really to the foot of the cross in a time of great need, or at any other time if it comes to that, means a great emptying out of self. Bereavement teaches that lesson of self-emptying. The self-sufficiency of daily life has been torn aside, the props of 'normality' are gone, the words 'man that is born of woman has but a short time to live . . .' become stark reality, not a flowery phrase from an archaic Prayer Book. Now, if ever, a man may go to the foot of the cross, and walk forward from it into the future carrying a cross. For that also is the lesson—to walk through life carrying one's own cross: joyfully, not in the ghastly subjection suggested by dismal pietists who talk about having to bear their crosses, but joyfully.

This is the lesson of bereavement: that life is meaningless unless it is walked with Christ, and carrying a cross. Some people who call themselves Christians try to believe, and persuade others, that it does not mean this; and by so doing they devitalise their faith and crucify their Lord again and again. But those who do learn it will discover new dimensions in all of their living.

For it will mean knowing peaks of joy never experienced before: it will also mean heartache unknown to those who try to dodge the storms of life. It will mean discipline: self-discipline, that dirty word so much disliked these days. It will mean rebellion, resentment and anger against a Lord who says 'Go *this* way', when the world and myself say—'Go that!'

It will mean never again being an exclusive little island, never just 'me', because words like 'me' and 'mine' cannot exist for the real disciple of Christ. But it will also mean living with a vividness of life never known before. From the point of bereavement into an unknown, and almost certainly feared future, is a long, hard, sometimes dangerous, sometimes lonely journey when you take that path in the faith and company of Christ; but as someone who has tried it, and often failed upon it, I would claim emphatically that the way of the cross is the only way for anyone who wants to experience life as our Creator surely meant us to experience it.

No, I am no stranger to suffering, death and bereavement, either for myself or for others. And, like St Paul in his second letter to the Corinthians, I feel entitled to do what he called a little 'boasting', though that is scarcely the apposite word. During the Second World War I spent two and a half years in hospital and reached the threshold of death on several occasions: more to the point, I also saw many good friends suffer and die.

My brother, whom I hero-worshipped, was killed in that same war.

My first wife and I helped nurse my father until he died in 1949. It was a difficult death—from cancer.

We nursed my young sister-in-law until she died in 1955. It was a difficult death—from cancer.

We nursed my mother until she died in 1960. It was a difficult death—from cancer.

And in 1963 I watched that same wife with whom I had lived seventeen wonderful years of partnership and love collapse and die from a heart attack, in a matter of minutes.

I am no stranger to suffering or death and bereavement, and I have learned that it is the fear of all these which is their greatest ally. Remove the fear, and the power of these facts of life and death to warp the human spirit is gone. And complete removal of fear I find only possible through faith in a living God; through trust in a Christ who had a human body like mine. Who lived, suffered and died. And went on living.

Death holds no fears for me: that I must affirm and I think I have won the right to do so. And, not fearing death, I can equally affirm with all the power at my command that it is the right and destiny of every individual to fight against and resist death as long as it is possible and reasonable to resist it. Fatalism has no part at all in my creed. I may not be afraid of death, but I see no merit in sitting down and letting death take its course while the human spirit can still fight, and while the outcome of that fight holds out some hope, however uncertain, of future days or years in this mortality.

We owe it to God, who gave us this life, to fight for it. We owe it to our families, our loved ones, to make a fight for life even when dying would be far easier, and involve far less personal suffering. And we owe it to ourselves! Our whole dignity as intelligent beings demands it. Our future life in the living beyond death may be of unimaginable happiness and bliss: it may be many things, but in this human state our minds cannot even begin to comprehend it. But we do know and understand this phase of life, even though our understanding is sometimes very sketchy, and I believe it is our task and duty to go on fighting for this life while there is the will and the reason to do so.

And this means that I go along with the doctors and surgeons who are slowly evolving the techniques of replacing worn-out parts of the human body with workable ones. Hard-line opponents of this school of medicine criticise the type of operation I have had on my heart. They question the morality of keeping my body alive artificially by means of a machine while the surgeon took the risk of cutting open my heart and replacing a couple of its unserviceable components. They ask whether it was not rather God's will that my natural span of time on this earth had come to an end, and I (and the surgeon) should have allowed death to foreclose on me. They query whether a man should walk about, live, breathe, drive a car, make love to his wife—do all the natural things to which I am now returning, with vital parts of the heart with which I was born gone, and man-made bits of metal doing their job instead.

The critics of replacement surgery query many things, but rarely do they seem to ask themselves what it can be like to look death bang in the eye—and then make a fight for life. A few weeks as a patient in an intensive-care cardiac unit might make them criticise and query less, and marvel more.

I have commented how sobering was the realisation of the fragility of the tightrope across which I had walked during and after my operation. Let me elaborate a little on that statement, for it has much bearing on the views I have just been expressing. During my eight weeks in that cardiac unit three patients were operated on for double-valve replacement: the same two valves in each case (the other two men prepared for open-heart surgery with me in our room in C3 were not of this trio). All of us were seriously ill; none of us had even a reasonable expectancy of life in our similar conditions of extreme heart impairment. Each one of us had had the risks of our particular type of advised surgery explained to us in detail by the medical team. None of us went forward to our operation unaware of what we, our families and the cardiac team were undertaking. Three of us, and each one understood the situation clearly. Each one knew that death was very near, and each one of us, as I found out later on, was a practising Christian.

Only one of those three survived: myself. Sobering? I can only repeat what I have said before: that I have never experienced humility, that most elusive of feelings, more deeply.

It was the right of each one of us, and of our families, to take the decision to undergo heart surgery. No pressure was put on any of us: on the contrary the decision was ours, and ours alone. Well aware of the risks in our individual cases (and the risks for no two people are ever exactly the same), we took them. Two died, and one survived, but if the same circumstances presented themselves to me again—then I would accept the risks again, and pit the skill of a cardiac team, my own will to live, and the prayers of my family and friends against all the armoury of suffering and death.

It is so immensely worth while accepting the challenge, because if one wins through then one is aware of a modern miracle having been performed in one's own body. And the whole quality of life and living steps into a higher key.

One last word must be said about cardiac surgeons and their teams before I quit ward A3—I trust for good.

My experience of cardiac units is confined to one hospital serving one area of the Midlands. Yet from what I have learnt since I left that hospital, the unit which fought my battle differs little from cardiac units in cities in many parts of the country. The same immense attention to detail is general. The same demanding standards of skill and technical proficiency. The same determination that a bond of understanding shall exist between the people who have to perform the surgery and see to the aftercare, and the person who puts him or herself into their hands. The same sadness and despondency when a patient for whom the team has fought so hard dies. The same compassion.

For this is part of the message I would try to convey to other people with severely damaged hearts, other patients now walking the road which may lead in the end to open-heart surgery.

Walk that road with confidence! The standard of skills and caring in this field of medicine, in this country, are second to none in the world. Other countries may publicise their achievements more widely. A few British people may struggle to raise money they can ill afford to have heart surgery performed in one or another of those perhaps more flamboyant countries. But they do the doctors and surgeons of this country less than justice.

Cardiac surgery in Britain is tremendously skilled, and if it is approached by most cardiac teams with a goodly dollop of British caution—so much the better. This is no field in which to take unnecessary chances: the risks attendant upon operating on the heart of a critically ill patient are big enough in all conscience. You, the heart-patient reading these words, can approach open-heart surgery without any fears for the skills, caution and compassion of your cardiac team. And even though the choices facing you—a brief period of living like a cabbage until heart failure ends your mortal journey, or accepting heart surgery with whatever attendant risks it holds for you—even though you are faced with an agonising Hobson's choice, you can be assured that the modern cardiac teams scattered throughout the hospitals of Britain do spell hope!

A footnote, then I am done with hospitals. So often criticised, so rarely given tribute for the magnificent work of caring it does—I refer to the often-abused Welfare State in which we live. Accept that there are loopholes in it, bureaucratic bunglings, inadequacies. It still enables any person in the land to have hospital treatment which would cost a small fortune in many another country.

One day a few weeks after my operation a fellow-patient and I, with the assistance of a knowledgeable sister, tried to work out what it would have cost me to have the treatment I had received, first as a private patient in Britain, secondly in an American hospital. On the first count we discovered that the sum total of all the national insurance stamps I have ever paid in my working life would come nowhere near covering the cost of surgeon's fees, cardiologist's fees, anaesthetist's fees, hospital bed and board, and the Lord knows what-all. And in America? Possibly by selling my house and car and everything I possess I might just have managed it. Possibly. I would not have been able to lie in a hospital bed week after week as I did in the Walsgrave—and not have to worry once where the money was coming from for all the skilled treatment I was getting. That is one of the facts of life of our criticised Welfare State. It is a pity it is not publicly recognised a little more often.

And the second part of the message I would try to share with those facing open-heart surgery?

It is very simple. Even a little faith in God—a power outside and bigger than oneself, a power whom millions still believe created us—even a shred of faith in the God of compassion and healing is a major weapon in the battle against suffering, and the fear of death. Any amount of faith need not prevent death from intervening. Why should it: faith is no insurance policy. But it does help one to face the basic issues of life calmly and with a quiet mind. And a quiet mind is probably the greatest aid both patient and surgeon can have when it comes to operating on the heart.

Even at the darkest period after my own operation, when my body was helpless and my mind clouded, I knew with certainty two things. That the prayers of a host of people were willing me to live. And that the Christ I had asked to come with me in those last seconds before the anaesthetic swamped everything, had done just that.

And I lived.

POST(OP) SCRIPT

This morning I stood on the summit of Hafod-y-boeth.

It is only a little mountain; in fact it cannot be truly classified as a mountain at all, its bracken and gorse-covered head falling well short of the qualifying one thousand feet. And I cannot claim to have walked all the way up its gentle ridges and cwms to reach the crest; the car which carried me most of the way stood in clear view on the winding road only a few hundred feet distant. But that final stretch of uneven upward scramble I did on my own feet; and as I stood on the top of that green Welsh hill I felt a sense of triumph which I doubt could be greater in any of the giants of the climbing world at last standing on the top of Everest.

Almost due north lay the cloud-capped head of Snowdon. South-west of me white-capped waves caught the fitful sunshine which defiantly broke through the cloud-wrack over Tremadoc Bay. Westwards, almost twenty miles away, the lesser peaks of the Lleyn Peninsula could be glimpsed beyond the Vale of Ffestiniog; and eastwards, as far as the eye could see, peaks and valleys rose and fell until they faded into the overcast. Way beyond them lay the border with England; and further still, a good hundred and fifty miles away, stood the hospital in which just nine months ago I walked down a very different valley from those which lay before me today.

Beside me on the top of Hafod-y-boeth stood Jo, a cautious ear cocked towards my rapidly clicking valves, but with a look on her face which I wish could have been seen by other wives or husbands facing the prospect of sweating out the vigil of open-heart surgery on their partners. Running wild through the tangled undergrowth of the ridge, Jonathan and Rebecca shouted and tumbled with the joy of puppies let off the leash, careless of the sweeping views, steeped in the heady wine of unpolluted air and a damp, cool wind almost blowing them off their feet.

And beside us, as staunch and reliable as they have always been, stood Pat and Christopher. Together we had shared the long pull up to, through, and away from the operation. Now, still together, we stood in a little group on the summit of a Welsh hill and shared—achievement I think is the word, although joy, triumph and sheer delight, in just being, all came into it. And worship. Unexpressed and unsaid; but felt, I believe, by each one of us.

In two weeks' time I am due to see the cardiologist again, and I will confess I have broken the rules by climbing my mini-mountain. But I think he will understand. And I think he will not be displeased when the slow, steady, even beating of my heart travels up his stethoscope. Because the rapid clicking on the hilltop this morning subsided to a true normal as swiftly as did the non-metallic hearts of my companions. True, my bones have taken a singularly poor view of the whole exercise; but as I sit and write in this remote cottage in Northern Wales, with not the noise of a car or plane or anything mechanical for miles to break the stillness, the only sound in this warm room is the slow, regular clicking from my man-made valves. And that slow clicking is the music of life.

It has not been an easy nine months, and the slog from my bed in A3 has been slow and demanding on both body and mind. When I left the Walsgrave in November I blithely imagined I could now forge ahead on a rapid return to normality. I really should have taken more notice of the cardiac team who stressed and re-stressed that it would all take a long time. The euphoria of returning home vanished with a crash as I was whisked back into hospital at Warwick just five days after saying goodbye to the Walsgrave. I was taking a high dose of anti-coagulants—would have to take them for the rest of my life—and my particular anti-clog pills decided to run amok. Covered in a maddening itchy rash from head to foot I was dumped in a ward at Warwick Hospital and the blood-letting began again while a different anti-coagulant was cautiously tried on me. For three days I sat in bed, glaring about the ward, and being insufferable to the doctors who I considered, and said, were taking caution to the slowest of slow extremes. With the blood-clotting factor in my blood still far too high they reluctantly let me go at the end of the three days, with strict instructions to report at the blood clinic twice a week until they had my blood, and the new anti-coagulant dose, stabilised. So I returned home, this time to stay there.

For a month I slept downstairs, drawing every last dram of pleasure from my home, my family and my friends, all the time trying to come to terms with the tiredness and weakness which still held me strongly in their grip. And, more than anything, trying to ignore the constant rapid, dominating clicking in my chest. At the end of the month I was allowed to go upstairs to sleep, and both surgeon and cardiologist expressed themselves pleased at the way things were progressing. But the heart-rate still remained far too high, zooming to ridiculous peaks at the slightest exertion. The weeks went by, then the months, and any signs of real health and strength coming my way seemed few. So the routine went on: rest, rest, and yet more rest, until I was heartily sick of the sound of the word.

The change came at the end of March, and it came swiftly. My heartbeat steadied from a gallop to a canter, from a canter to a trot, from a trot to—this which I can hear now as I write. A slow, regular, life-giving beat. Strength began invading my body, and slowly, cautiously, I became more active. Work was still banned, but I began to get out and about, began to walk without exhaustion interfering. I was able to play with the children again and, above all, I started being able to ignore for hours, even days on end, the mechanical clicking from my chest. Still the cardiologist stressed the need to rest, and I heeded him. I knew now that the tide had turned and I had no desire to go back to square one.

Now it is the end of June in this drop-out summer of 1972. For almost a week we have been exploring old haunts, and despite the rain and wind and a temperature which would disgrace February, the views have seemed wider, the mountains higher, the grass greener, the magic of Wales stronger than ever.

And this morning I climbed to the top of Hafod-y-boeth.

The others had no difficulty in keeping ahead of me as we wound our way up the slopes. They waited cheerfully during my frequent halts to gulp air down into my hard-working lungs. They tactfully did not enquire how my hip and legs were enjoying this latest caper: in retrospect I imagine they did not want a flow of bad language to sully the clean air on that Welsh hillside. And they stood on the summit waiting for me to join them—but they had better watch out!

It is not beyond the bounds of possibility that, given time, I might get that new hip: I can at least start twisting the arm of the cardiologist about it. And then I may even be able to beat my beloved Jo, my children and these dearest of friends to the top of the mountain. Although, whether I do or not matters little: the views from the top will be still wide, and still beckoning.

And no one walks into that land on the other side of the mountain alone.